# PÖCKET
# PASSED
## NURSE PRACTITIONER

Lauren Knobeloch, ACNP, FNP

i

© 2020 Pocket Pimped, LLC
www.PocketPassed.com
ISBN: 978-1-7343287-3-8

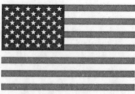

Printed in the United States of America

# Specialty Contributors

**Kate Becker, MSN, APN, FNP-BC, ACNPC-AG**
New Lenox, IL

**Sherri Bissell, MSN, FNP-C, ENP-C**
Charlotte, NC

**Jordan Clayton, MSN, APRN, FNP-BC, AOCNP**
Charlotte, NC

**Courtney DuBois Shihabuddin, DNP, APRN-CNP**
Columbus, OH

**Rose Grady, FNP-C**
Columbus, OH

**Corinna Hughes, DNP, FNP-C**
Rochester, MN

**Andrea M. Kurtz, FNP-C**
Charlotte, NC

**Danielle LeVeck, DNP, ACNPC-AG, CCNS, CCRN, RN**
Cleveland, OH

# Specialty Contributors

**Allie McAllister, NP-C, DCNP**
Atlanta, GA

**Steve Rieke, AGNP, DNP**
Rochester, MN

**Martha A. Roberts, MSN, ACNP, PNP, BSN, CEN, CPEN**
Sacramento, CA

**Elizabeth Rohr, MSN, FNP-BC**
Boston, MA

**Elizabeth Russ MSN, FNP-C**
State College, PA

**Shirley A. Triplet, MSN, NP-BC**
Buffalo, NY

**Heather L. Truchelut, FNP-BC, NP-C**
Paterson, NJ

To my very supportive and loving husband, who keeps me laughing every day. You are the most incredible husband and father to our children.

To my amazing children, who I love and adore more than words. Being your mom will always be my greatest blessing.

You are my world, and I love you!

# Contents

**Health Maintenance**       **1**

I.    Types of Prevention .......................... 2

II.   Statistical Tests .............................. 2

III.   Screening .................................... 3

- Abdominal Aortic Aneurysm (AAA)
- Breast Cancer
- Cervical Cancer & HPV
- Colorectal Cancer
- Diabetes Mellitus
- High Blood Pressure
- Sexually Transmitted Infections
- Human Immunodeficiency Virus (HIV)
- Hepatitis C
- Lipid Disorder
- Osteoporosis & Osteopenia
- Prostate Cancer
- Lung Cancer
- Skin Cancer
- Obesity
- Newborn

IV.   Vaccinations ............................... 9

- Live Attenuated Virus Vaccine
- Tetanus
- Human Papillomavirus (HPV)
- Meningitis
- Shingles

- Pneumonia
- Measles, Mumps, Rubella (MMR)
- Hepatitis B
- Influenza
- Varicella
- Rotavirus

## Cardiovascular System 17

I. General Cardiology ......................................................18
II. Hypertensions ..........................................................19
III. Hypotension & Shock ...............................................23
IV. Hyperlipidemia ........................................................25
V. Cardiomyopathy ........................................................26
- Dilated Cardiomyopathy
- Hypertrophic Cardiomyopathy
- Restrictive Cardiomyopathy

VI. Coronary Artery Disease ..........................................28
VII. Valvular Disorders ..................................................32
VIII. Conduction Disorders & Dysrhythmias .....34
- Atrial fibrillation (AF)
- Sinus Bradycardia
- Heart Block
- Supraventricular Dysrhythmias
- Ventricular Dysrhythmias

IX. Heart Failure ............................................................39
X. Heart Inflammation ...................................................42
- Pericarditis
- Endocarditis

XI. Congenital Heart Disease .........................................45

XII. Vascular Diseases ............................ 46
- Aortic Aneurysms
- Limb Ischemia
- Peripheral Artery Disease (PAD)
- Venous Thromboses
- Deep Vein Thrombosis (DVT)
- Chronic Venous Insufficiency

## Pulmonary System    53

I.   General Pulmonology ............................ 54
II.  Pulmonary Infections ............................ 56
- Pneumonia
- Tuberculosis
- Bronchiolitis
- Bronchitis
- Croup
- Epiglottitis
- Influenza
- Pertussis
III. Obstructive Airway Disease ............................ 63
- COPD
- Asthma
IV. Restrictive Lung Disease ............................ 67
- Cystic Fibrosis
- Sarcoidosis
- Idiopathic Pulmonary Fibrosis
V.  Pleural Disease ............................ 68
- General
- Pleural Effusion

- Pneumothorax
VI.  Pulmonary Circulation ............................ 71
- Pulmonary Embolism
- Pulmonary Hypertension
- Cor Pulmonale
VII. Neoplasms ............................................ 75
VIII. Sleep Apnea ......................................... 76
IX.  ARDS ................................................... 77

## Gastrointestinal System      79

I.   General Gastroenterology ...................... 80
II.  Small Intestine Disorders ...................... 81
- Celiac Disease
- Appendicitis
- Intussusception
- Small Bowel Obstruction (SBO)
- Volvulus
- Ileus
III. Biliary Disorders ................................... 85
- Cholecystitis
IV.  Colorectal Disorders .............................. 87
- Diverticulosis
- Inflammatory Bowel Disease (IBD)
V.   Colorectal Cancer .................................. 90
VI.  Constipation ......................................... 91
VII. Hemorrhoids ......................................... 91
VIII. Anal Fissure ......................................... 92
IX.  Anorectal Fistula .................................... 92

X. Irritable Bowel Syndrome (IBS) .............. 93

XI. Mesenteric Ischemia ........................ 93

XII. Large Bowel Obstruction .................. 94

XIII. Esophageal Disorders ..................... 95

- GERD
- Esophagitis
- Barrett Esophagus
- Mallory-Weiss Tears
- Esophageal Varices

XIV. Gastric Disorders ......................... 98

- Gastritis
- Peptic Ulcer Disease
- Pyloric Stenosis

XV. Hepatic Disorders .......................... 99

- Hepatitis
- Nonalcoholic Fatty Liver Disease (NAFLD)
- Ascites
- Acute Liver Failure
- Portal Hypertension

XVI. Pancreatic Disorders ..................... 102

- Acute Pancreatitis

XVII. Hernias ................................. 104

XVIII. Infectious Diarrhea .................... 104

- Gastroenteritis
- Clostridium Difficile (C. Diff)

XIX. Miscellaneous ........................... 105

## Endocrine System     107

   I.    Diabetes Mellitus _____108
   II.   Thyroid Disorders _____111
- Hypothyroidism
- Hyperthyroidism
- Thyroiditis

  III.  Adrenal Disorders _____115
- Adrenal Insufficiency
- Pheochromocytoma

  IV.  Parathyroid Disorders _____118
   V.   Pituitary Disorders _____119
  VI.  Diabetes Insipidus _____120


## Dermatologic System     121

   I.    Acneiform Eruptions _____122
   II.   Desquamation _____123
  III.  Hair & Nails _____124
  IV.  Exanthems _____124
   V.   Infectious Diseases _____125
  VI.  Neoplasms _____127
 VII.  Papulosquamous Disorders _____128
VIII.  Skin Integrity _____129
  IX.  Other Dermatologic Disorders _____130
   X.   Pediatrics _____133


## Eyes, Ears, Nose & Throat     137

   I.    Eye Disorders _____138
- Conjunctivitis

- Cataracts
- Corneal Ulcer (Keratitis)
- Herpes Simplex Keratitis
- Pterygium/Pinguecula
- Lacrimal Glands
- Blepharitis
- Chalazion/Hordeolum
- Nystagmus
- Papilledema
- Orbital Cellulitis
- Macular Degeneration
- Retinal Detachment
- Retinopathy
- Orbital Fracture
- Corneal Abrasion
- Ruptured Globe
- Hyphema
- Subconjunctival Hemorrhage
- Uveitis
- Central Retinal Artery/Vein Occlusion
- Amaurosis Fugax
- Amblyopia
- Glaucoma
- Strabismus
- Optic Neuritis
- Foreign Bodies
- Retinoblastoma
- Miscellaneous

II. Ear Disorders ........................................ 151
- Cerumen Impaction

- Otitis Externa
- Malignant Otitis Externa
- Otitis Media
- Subperichondrial Hematoma
- Foreign Bodies
- Barotrauma
- Ruptured Tympanic Membrane
- Eustachian Tube Dysfunction
- Labyrinthitis
- Vertigo
- Presbycusis
- Mastoiditis
- Meniere's Disease
- Tinnitus

III. Nose & Sinus Disorders _____ 157
- Epistaxis
- Allergic Rhinitis
- Sinusitis
- Foreign Bodies

IV. Oropharyngeal Disorders _____ 159
- Dental Abscess
- Vincent's Angina
- Aphthous Ulcers
- Oral Candidiasis
- Leukoplakia
- HSV-1
- Laryngitis
- Peritonsillar Abscess
- Pharyngitis
- Sialadenitis

- Parotitis

## Genitourinary System     165

I.   Incontinence _____166
- General
- Urge Incontinence
- Stress Incontinence
- Mixed Incontinence
- Overflow Incontinence
- Functional/Transient Incontinence

II.   Overactive Bladder _____168

III.  Infectious Disorders _____168
- Cystitis
- Pyelonephritis
- Urethritis
- Epididymitis
- Orchitis
- Prostatitis
- Fournier Gangrene

IV.  Neoplasms _____171
- Bladder Cancer
- Penile Cancer
- Prostate Cancer
- Testicular Cancer

V.   Nephrolithiasis/Urolithiasis _____173

VI.  Urethral Disorders _____174

VII. Penile Disorders _____175
- Erectile Dysfunction
- Epispadias/Hypospadias

- Priapism
- Peyronie's Disease
- Phimosis/Paraphimosis
- Balanitis

VIII. Benign Prostatic Hyperplasia ............ 177
IX.  Testicular Disorders ............................ 177
- Hydrocele/Varicocele
- Testicular Torsion
- Cryptorchidism

## Reproductive System      181

I.    Breast Disorders ............................... 182
II.   Cervical Disorders ............................ 183
III.  Complicated Pregnancy .................... 183
IV.   Contraceptive Methods ..................... 188
V.    Menopause ........................................ 189
VI.   Menstrual Disorders ......................... 189
VII.  Neoplasms ........................................ 191
VIII. Ovarian Disorders ............................ 192
IX.   Sexual Transmitted Infections & Pelvic
      Inflammatory Disease ....................... 193
X.    Trauma ............................................. 195
XI.   Uncomplicated Pregnancy ................ 195
XII.  Uterine Disorders ............................. 198
XIII. Vaginal & Vulvar Disorders ............. 198
XIV.  Miscellaneous ................................... 199

# Neurologic System     201

I. Headaches ..................................................... 202
- Migraines
- Cluster Headaches
- Tension Headaches
- Trigeminal Neuralgia
- Idiopathic Intracranial Hypertension
- Red Flag Symptoms

II. Closed Head Injuries ................................. 205

III. Cranial Nerve Palsies ............................... 206

IV. Encephalopathic Disorders ...................... 207
- Encephalopathy
- Reye Syndrome

V. Infectious Disorders ................................. 209
- Encephalitis & Meningitis

VI. Movement Disorders ............................... 211
- Essential Tremors
- Huntington Disease
- Parkinson Disease

VII. Neurocognitive Disorders ..................... 211
- Delirium, Dementia, & Alzheimer's Disease

VIII. Neuromuscular Disorders ..................... 213
- Cerebral Palsy
- Multiple Sclerosis
- Myasthenia Gravis
- ALS (Lou Gehrig's Disease)

IX. Peripheral Nerve Disorders .................... 214
- Carpal Tunnel Syndrome
- Guillain-Barre Syndrome

- Diabetic Neuropathy
- Bell's Palsy

X.  Seizure Disorders ................................. 217
- General
- Absence Seizures
- Febrile Seizures
- Status Epilepticus

XI.  Vascular Disorders ................................. 219
- Cerebral Aneurysms & Hemorrhage
- Stroke & TIA
- Giant Cell Arteritis (GCA)

XII. Miscellaneous ................................. 223
- Reflexes
- Neoplasms
- Vertigo
- Abuse

## Hematologic System    227

I.    Idiopathic Thrombocytopenic Purpura ... 228
II.   Coagulation Disorders ......................... 228
III.  Thrombocytopenia ................................. 229
IV.  Cytopenias ................................. 231
- General
- Hemolytic Anemia
- Macrocytic Anemia
- Normocytic Anemia
- Microcytic Anemia

V.    Cytoses ................................. 236
- Polycythemia Vera

- Essential Thrombocytopenia
VI. Hemoglobinopathies _____ 238
- Diagnosis
- Hemochromatosis
- Sickle Cell Disease
- Thalassemia
VII. Neoplasms _____ 239
- Leukemias
- Multiple Myeloma
- Hodgkin's & Non-Hodgkin's Lymphoma

## Infectious Disease     243

I. Bacterial Diseases _____ 244
- Botulism
- Diphtheria
- Gonococcal
- MRSA
- S. Pneumoniae
- Rheumatic Fever
- Rocky Mountain Spotted Fever
- Tetanus
II. Fungal Diseases _____ 248
- Candidal Infections
III. Mycobacterium Avium Complex _____ 248
IV. Parasitic Diseases _____ 249
- Pinworms
- Malaria
- Giardia
V. Prenatal Transmission of Disorders _____ 250

VI.  Spirochetal Diseases .................... 251
- Lyme Disease
- Syphilis

VII. Viral Diseases .................... 252
- Infectious Mononucleosis
- HIV/AIDS
- Influenza
- Measles, Mumps, Rubella (MMR)
- Erythema Infectiosum
- Roseola
- Rabies
- Varicella Zoster
- Rotavirus
- Norovirus
- Zika

VIII. Systemic Inflammatory Response
Syndrome (SIRS) & Sepsis .................... 258

## Renal System                                261

I.   Acute Disorders .................... 262
- General
- Glomerulonephritis
- Hemolytic Uremic Syndrome
- Lupus Nephritis

II.  Acute Kidney Injury .................... 264

III. Chronic Kidney Disease .................... 265

IV.  Congenital & Structural Disorders ........ 267
- Polycystic Kidney Disease
- Renal Artery Stenosis

V.   End-Stage Renal Disease......268
VI.  Fluid & Electrolyte Disorders......269
  • General
  • SIADH

## Musculoskeletal System — 277

I.    Chest & Rib Disorders......278
II.   Compartment Syndrome......278
III.  Osteoarthritis......279
IV.   Osteoporosis......280
V.    Rickets......281
VI.   Infectious Diseases......281
  • Osteomyelitis
  • Septic Joint
  • Tenosynovitis
VII.  Upper Extremity Disorders......283
  • Clavicle
  • Shoulder
  • Elbow
  • Forearm
  • Hand & Wrist
VIII. Lower Extremity Disorders......287
  • Hip
  • Pelvis
  • Knee
  • Foot & Ankle
IX.   Neoplasms......293
X.    Rheumatologic Disorders......294
  • Systemic Lupus Erythematosus (SLE)

- Rheumatoid Arthritis (RA)
- Sjogren's Syndrome
- Polymyalgia Rheumatica
- Reactive Arthritis
- Raynaud's Syndrome
- Gout
- Fibromyalgia

XI. Spinal Disorders................................298

## Healthcare Policy & Ethics ............ 303

I. General..............................................304

# Preface

As a Nurse Practitioner with over a decade of experience, I have completed clinical rotations, the national board certification, the recertification process, and numerous continuing education courses. Throughout my career I have struggled to find a high-yield resource that is comprehensive, yet concise. This led to the creation of *Pocket Passed: Nurse Practitioner*. Working together with *Pocket Pimped* and other Nurse Practitioner educators from throughout the United States, we have created a book specifically designed for you! This text represents everything we are as medical providers: passionate, professional, and knowledgeable. We hope this resource serves useful to you and we wish you all the best in your pursuits.

# HEALTH
# MAINTENANCE

# *Types of Prevention*

1. What are the three types of prevention?
   - Primary prevention: Measures taken to prevent injury and promote health *before* the disease process begins (ie. immunizations, regular exercise, bike helmet safety)
   - Secondary prevention: Focuses on early detection *and* treatment of an existing disease or injury (ie. mammograms, prostate cancer screening)
   - Tertiary prevention: Rehabilitation and recovery (ie. physical therapy, cardiac rehabilitation, support groups (like Alcoholic Anonymous)
2. What is the incidence rate?
   - Number of new cases during a specified period of time divided by the number of people at risk
3. What is the prevalence rate?
   - Number of existing cases at a point in time divided by total number of people in the population

# *Statistical Tests*

4. What does the sensitivity of a test indicate?
   - True positive rate
5. What does the specificity of a test indicate?
   - True negative rate

# *Screening*

From the USPSTF Guidelines

## *Abdominal Aortic Aneurysm (AAA)*

6. What is the recommend screening tool for AAA? Who should be screened?

> ➢ Abdominal Ultrasound
> ➢ One-time screening for men ages 65-75 who have ever smoked

## *Breast Cancer*

7. At what age is breast cancer screening with mammography recommended in women of average risk? How often should screening occur?

> ➢ 50-74 years old
> ➢ Every other year
> ▪ Site source: USPSTF

8. What are some risk factors associated with breast cancer?

> ➢ Age ≥50, female, white race, family history, genetic mutations, obesity, endogenous estrogen and hormone therapy, nulliparity, increased age at time of first pregnancy, early menarche, late menopause, personal history of breast cancer

## *Cervical Cancer & HPV*

9. At what age should women undergo cervical cancer screening?

> ➢ 21-65 years old

10. What are the two primary tests used for cervical cancer screening?

> Pap smear for cervical cytology and HPV DNA

11. At what age should HPV DNA testing be considered for cervical cancer screening?

> ≥30 years old

12. What is the screening interval for Pap smears in women 21-29 years old? Women 30-65 years old?

> 21-29 years old: Every 3 years for Pap smear only with a normal prior result
> 30-69 years old: Every 5 years for Pap smear plus HPV DNA negative results

## *Colorectal Cancer*

13. What are the screening tools used to help detect colorectal cancer?

> High-sensitivity Fecal Occult Blood Test (FOBT) yearly
> Sigmoidoscopy every 5 years
> Colonoscopy every 10 years
> Cologuard (DNA fit) every 1-3 years
> FIT every year

14. What are risk factors for colorectal cancer?

> Family history, inflammatory bowel disease (ie. ulcerative colitis, Chron's disease), African American race, male sex, smoker, obesity, alcohol consumption

## *Diabetes Mellitus*

15. Which patients should be screened for type 2 diabetes mellitus?
> Age >40 years if overweight or obese, history of gestational DM, everyone age >45 years, first degree relative with DM, those with HTN and/or PCOS, history of CVD

## *High Blood Pressure*

16. How should screening of hypertension be obtained and on which patients?
> Office blood pressure measurements should be checked on all patients ≥18 years old
> Obtaining blood pressure readings outside of the clinical setting for diagnostic confirmation is recommended prior to starting treatment

## *Sexually Transmitted Infections*

17. When should patients be screened for chlamydia and gonorrhea?
- Sexually active women ≤24 years old
- In women >24 years old who are at increased risk for infection
- Men who have sex with men (MSM)

## *Human Immunodeficiency Virus (HIV)*

18. When should patients be screened for HIV?
> Age 15-65
> Young adolescents and adults at increased risk

> All pregnant women
>   - Including laboring women or at time of delivery is HIV status is unknown

19. What is PrEP?
> Pre-exposure prophylaxis with effective antiretroviral therapy
>   - Should be offered to patients at high risk of acquiring HIV

20. Which individuals are considered high risk for HIV?
> Men who have sex with men
> IV drug users
> Transgender women

21. How often should at risk individuals be screened for HIV?
>   - Yearly
>   - After a known high-risk exposure

## Hepatitis C

22. The USPSTF recommends screening for hepatitis C virus infection for what age group of patients?
> Adults 18-79 years old

## Lipid Disorder

23. What are the 3 criteria that if all are met the USPSTF recommends use of low to moderate-dose statin to help prevent CVD event and morality?
> Age 40-75
> ≥1 CVD risk factors (ie. dyslipidemia, DM, HTN, or smoking)

> Calculated 10-year risk of a cardiovascular event of ≥10%

## Osteoporosis & Osteopenia

24. When should women be screened for osteoporosis with a DEXA scan?
    > Women ≥65 years old
    > Postmenopausal women <65 years old with high-risk factors for osteoporosis as determined by a formal clinical risk assessment tool

## Prostate Cancer

25. What are some risk factors for Prostate Cancer?
    > Increased age
      - Especially >65 years old
    > African American race
    > Family history of prostate cancer
26. When is prostate cancer screening indicated?
    > For men 55-69 years old (USPSTF) or 50 years old (ACS)
      - However, the decision should be based on shared decision making with the patient as there are no societal recommendations for hard set indications for screening

## Lung Cancer

27. What screening tool is used to detect lung cancer? Which patients should be screened?
    > Annual screening with low-dose computed tomography (LDCT)

- Site source: USPSTF
➢ Adults aged 50-80 years with a 20 pack-year smoking history & currently smoke or quit within the past 15 years

28. When can lung cancer screening be discontinued?
➢ Once a patient has not smoked for 15 years
➢ Patient develops a health problem that ultimately limits life expectancy or the ability/willingness to have a curative lung surgery

29. How do you calculate a patient's pack-year smoking history?
➢ Number of packs of cigarettes smoked per day multiplied by the number of years the patient has smoked

## Skin Cancer

30. When should counseling about minimizing exposure to ultraviolet (UV) radiation occur?
➢ Age 6 months to 24 years
- Especially with fair skin types

## Obesity

31. When should clinicians offer or refer a patient for intensive, multicomponent behavioral interventions?
➢ BMI ≥30 kg/m²

32. What BMI range is defined as underweight? Normal weight? Overweight? Obese class I? Obese class II? Obese class III?
➢ Underweight: <18.5 kg/m²
➢ Normal weight: ≥18.5 to 24.9 kg/m²

➤ Overweight: ≥25.0 to 29.9 kg/m²
➤ Obese class I: 30.0 to 34.9 kg/m²
➤ Obese class II: 35.0 to 39.9 kg/m²
➤ Obese class III: ≥40 kg/m²

33. Which types of cancers does the USPSTF not recommend routine screening for?

➤ Ovarian Cancer
➤ Prostate Cancer
➤ Testicular Cancer
➤ Oral Cancer
➤ Pancreatic Cancer

### Newborn

34. What percentage of birth weight may term newborns lose in the first 5-7 days of life? When should this weight be regained?

➤ Up to 10%
➤ Within 10-14 days of life

## Vaccinations

### Live Attenuated Virus Vaccine

35. What is a live attenuated virus vaccine?

➤ Vaccines that contain bacteria or viruses which are weakened compared to the natural disease in order to help the body produce an immune response

36. What are common live attenuated vaccines that should be avoided in immunocompromised patients?

➤ Varicella

> Measles, mumps, rubella (MMR)
> Live attenuated influenza vaccine

## *Tetanus*

37. When do you administer tetanus toxoid containing vaccine with or without tetanus immunoglobulins?

> ≥3 lifetime tetanus toxoid doses
>   - Clean or minor wound: Tetanus toxoid vaccine only if the last dose was ≥10 years prior
>   - Dirty or severe or "all other" wounds: Tetanus toxoid vaccine only if the last dose was ≥5 years prior
> Unimmunized, uncertain, or <3 tetanus toxoid lifetime doses
>   - Clean or minor wound: Tetanus toxoid containing vaccine only
>   - Dirty or severe or "all other" wounds: Tetanus toxoid containing vaccine AND tetanus immunoglobulins
> Persons who have HIV or are severely immunocompromised with a contaminated wound should receive human tetanus immunoglobin regardless of tetanus vaccination history

38. What are the routine tetanus, diphtheria, and pertussis (Tdap) vaccination recommendations in immunocompetent patients?

> All pregnant women between 27-36 weeks gestation for EVERY pregnancy

> Tetanus and diphtheria toxin (Td) booster every
> 10 years for all adults with a one-time Tdap
> vaccine in lieu of Td

## *Human Papillomavirus (HPV)*

39. When should the HPV vaccine be administered in
immunocompetent individuals?

> Men and women 11-12 years old (may be
> initiated as early as 9 years old)
>   - If not obtained by 12 years old, vaccine may be
>     given up to 26 years old
>   - May consider vaccine up to 46 years old in
>     patients that may benefit

40. What are the indications for a two-dose and three-
dose schedule for HPV vaccination?

> Two-dose schedule: Recommended for patients
> that receive their first dose prior to their 15th
> birthday, and the second dose 6-12 months after
> the first dose
> Three-dose schedule: Recommended for patients
> who get the first dose on or after their 15th
> birthday, or (2) have certain
> immunocompromised conditions, or (3) if a
> second dose was administered before a 5-month
> interval from the first dose

## *Meningitis*

41. What are the two types of meningococcal vaccines
available?

> Meningococcal conjugate vaccine

➢ Serogroup B meningococcal vaccine

42. When should the meningococcal conjugate vaccines be given?

➢ All patients 11-12 years old
➢ Booster dose given at age 16

43. Who should be considered for receiving serogroup B meningococcal vaccine?

➢ Adolescents and young adults (age 16-23 years old)
➢ Individuals at increased risk for developing meningitis (ie. college students living in dormitories, exposed patient, military recruits, asplenia, travels to endemic areas

## Shingles

44. Who should receive the shingles vaccine?

➢ Age ≥50 years old
➢ CDC recommends two doses of Zoster recombinant (ie. Shingrix) vaccine separated by 2 to 6 months for immunocompetent patients
➢ Give regardless of history of shingles

## Pneumonia

45. What are the two types of pneumococcal vaccines available in the United States?

➢ Pneumococcal conjugate vaccine (PCV13; Prevnar)
➢ Pneumococcal polysaccharide vaccine (PPSV23; Pneumovax)

46. What is the routine vaccine administration schedule for the pneumococcal vaccine?

> In patients 19-64 years old with a history of diabetes, alcoholism, cigarette smoking, chronic heart (excluding hypertension), lung, or liver disease: PPSV23 alone should be administered

  ▪ At age 65 these individuals should then receive PCV13 followed by another dose of PPSV23 at least 1 year from prior PCV13

> Patients 19-64 years old who are immunocompromised (ie. HIV, malignancy, nephrotic syndrome, solid organ transplant), CSF leaks, cochlear implants, sickle cell disease, iatrogenic immunosuppressive, asplenism, or CKD should receive sequential vaccination with PCV13 followed by PPSV23 8 weeks apart

  ▪ A subsequent dose of PPSV23 should be given at least 5 years thereafter (or at 65 years old)

## Measles, Mumps, Rubella (MMR)

47. What three diseases does the MMR vaccine protect against? When should the vaccine be administered?

> Measles, mumps, and rubella
> Two doses:
  ▪ 1st dose: 12-15 months old
  ▪ 2nd dose: 4-6 years old

## Hepatitis B

48. How many doses is the hepatitis B vaccine? When are they administered?

- Three doses
  - Given at birth, 1 month, and 6 months

49. When should screening for the hepatitis B virus occur? In which patients?
  - Adolescents and adults at increased risk
  - Pregnant women at 1st prenatal visit

## *Influenza*

50. What is the CDC recommendation for the influenza vaccine?
  - Annual vaccination for all patients who are ≥6 months old (who do not have contraindications)
    - 2 doses for first-time in patients 6 months to 8 years

## *Varicella*

51. What are some contraindications for the varicella vaccine?
  - Pregnancy, immunocompromised state (ie. HIV, leukemia), prolonged high dose immunosuppressive therapy (including large dose oral steroids), received blood products within last 3-11 months

## *Rotavirus*

52. What are the symptoms of rotavirus? What vaccines are available? When should the vaccine be administered?
  - Symptoms: severe watery diarrhea, vomiting, fever, abdominal pain

- Two vaccines available: RotaTeq (3 doses) and Rotarix (2 doses)
- 1st dose should be given before 15 weeks of age and the last dose prior to 8 months of age
  - Rotarix (RV1) is given in 2 doses at ages 2 months and 4 months
  - RotaTeq (RV5) is given in 3 doses at ages 2 months, 4 months, and 6 months

# Health Maintenance

**2**

---

# CARDIOVASCULAR SYSTEM

Cardiovascular System

## *General Cardiology*

53. How does blood flow through the heart?
    ➤ Blood enters the heart through the
      superior/inferior vena cava → right atrium →
      through the tricuspid valve → right ventricle →
      through the pulmonic valve → pulmonary artery
      → lung → pulmonary veins → left atrium →
      through the mitral valve → left ventricle →
      through the aortic valve → aorta → blood exits
      the heart to the body

54. Where is the Point of Maximal Impulse (PMI)
located? And what could displacement of PMI suggest?
    ➤ Location: 5th intercostal space at the
      midclavicular line
    ➤ Displacement may suggest LVH or enlargement

55. What are the levels of the Heart Murmur Grading
System?
    ➤ Grade I: Faintest, barely audible
    ➤ Grade II: Audible but soft murmur
    ➤ Grade III: Easily audible, moderate murmur, no
      palpable thrill
    ➤ Grade IV: Loud murmur, associated with
      palpable thrill
    ➤ Grade V: Very loud murmur, heard with placing
      stethoscope lightly on chest
    ➤ Grade VI: Extremely loud, audible with
      stethoscope off the chest

56. What is stroke volume?
    ➤ The volume of blood ejected from the heart

57. Stroke volume directly depends on what three properties?

> - Preload
> - Myocardial Contractility
> - Afterload

58. What are the three classifications of cardiomyopathy?

> - Dilated
> - Restrictive
> - Hypertrophic

## Hypertension

59. What are the 4 blood pressure categories for adults per the American Heart Association?

> - Normal: Systolic pressure <120 mmHg **AND** diastolic <80 mmHg
> - Elevated blood pressure: Systolic pressure of 120-129 mmHg and diastolic <80 mmHg
> - Stage I hypertension: Systolic pressure of 130-139 mmHg **OR** diastolic 80-89 mmHg
> - Stage II hypertension: Systolic pressure ≥140 mmHg **OR** diastolic ≥90 mmHg

60. What are the major organs affected by hypertension?

> - Brain, kidney, heart, & vascular systems

61. What is the most common cause of death in hypertensive patients?

> - Heart disease

62. What is the difference between primary and secondary hypertension?

> Primary – no specific identifiable cause
> Secondary – identifiable cause

63. What are the common causes of secondary hypertension?

> **C**ushing syndrome
> **H**yperaldosteronism
> **A**orta coarctation
> **P**heochromocytoma
> **S**tenosis of renal artery
  - Remember: "**CHAPS**"

64. What are lifestyle modifications used as nonpharmacologic therapy to treat HTN?

> DASH diet, salt restriction (maximum intake of 2.4g/day), weight reduction, exercise, limitation of alcohol intake, stress management, smoking cessation

65. What is the DASH Diet?

> "**D**ietary **A**pproaches to **S**top **H**ypertension"
> Diet rich in vegetables, fruits, low fat-dairy products
> Reduced saturated and total fat

66. What is the definition of white coat hypertension?

> Consistently elevated in-office blood pressure measurements with normal out-of-office blood pressure measurements that do not meet criteria for hypertension

67. What are the complications of long-standing uncontrolled hypertension?

> Heart failure (systolic and/or diastolic), ischemic heart disease, left ventricular hypertrophy,

ischemic or hemorrhagic stroke, retinopathy, chronic kidney disease

68. What are the 4 classes of medications that may be used as first line therapy in the management of hypertension?

> Angiotensin converting enzyme inhibitors (ACEi)
> Angiotensin receptor blockers (ARB)
> Thiazide diuretics
> Long acting (dihydropyridine) calcium channel blockers

69. What is the definition of drug-resistant hypertension?

> ≥3 antihypertensives at maximum dose (one of which is a diuretic)

70. What is the first line therapy for a patient with hypertension and chronic kidney disease (CKD)?

> ACEi/ARB

71. What is the first line therapy for hypertension in African American patients without CKD?

> Dihydropyridine calcium channel blocker or thiazide diuretic

72. What are some potential adverse side effects of ACE inhibitors?

> Cough, angioedema, hyperkalemia, hypotension

73. What are two common electrolyte abnormalities that can occur with thiazide diuretics?

> Hyponatremia, hypokalemia

74. What are the adverse side effects of calcium channel blockers?

> Headache, edema, constipation, hypotension

75. What is the difference between hypertensive urgency and hypertensive emergency?

> HTN Urgency: Severe hypertension, asymptomatic, no evidence of end-organ damage
> HTN Emergency: Severe hypertension with acute end-organ damage

76. What is the triad of symptoms for hypertensive encephalopathy?

> Severe hypertension
> Altered mental status
> Papilledema (often present)

77. What three medications are used to treat hypertensive encephalopathy?

> Nitroprusside
> Nicardipine
> Labetalol

78. Why should you avoid reducing the blood pressure too quickly in hypertensive emergency?

> It can cause ischemia in organs that have been habituated to higher levels of blood pressure

79. What are some medications that can elevate blood pressure or decrease the efficacy of antihypertensive medications?

> Oral contraceptives, NSAIDs, steroids, nasal decongestants, over-the-counter cough/cold medications, antidepressants

80. What are the three components of metabolic syndrome?

> Hypertension

➢ Dyslipidemia
➢ Insulin resistance

81. What does hypertension, proteinuria >1000mg/day, and active urine sediment indicate?

➢ Primary renal disease

82. What is a catecholamine-secreting tumor located in the adrenal medulla that causes hypertension called? What is the definitive treatment?

➢ Pheochromocytoma
➢ Surgical excision of tumor

83. What retinal changes are seen in long-standing hypertension?

➢ Arteriolar narrowing, arteriovenous compression, papilledema, retinal hemorrhages or exudates

## Hypotension & Shock

84. What is orthostatic hypotension? How is it defined?

➢ Hypotension provoked by changes in position
➢ >20 mmHg drop in systolic blood pressure or >10 mmHg drop in diastolic blood pressure within 3 minutes of standing

85. What is vasovagal hypotension? What are the common triggers?

➢ Transient drop in blood pressure due to sympathetic activity that leads to cerebral hypoperfusion and syncope
➢ Triggered by prolonged standing, stressful events, heat, straining

86. What are the symptoms of vasovagal hypotension?

> Narrowing vision, lightheadedness, palpitations, cold sweats, syncope

87. What are the four types of shock?
> Obstructive
> Cardiogenic
> Distributive
> Hypovolemic

88. What is the most common type of shock?
> Distributive shock

89. What is the least common type of shock?
> Obstructive shock

90. What is obstructive shock? What are some causes?
> Obstruction of the systemic or pulmonary circulation
> Causes: pulmonary embolism, pulmonary hypertension, cardiac tamponade, tension pneumothorax, high PEEP

91. What is distributive shock? What are some causes? Which cause is most common?
> Systemic vasodilation
> Sepsis (most common), anaphylaxis, neurogenic

92. What is cardiogenic shock? What are some causes? Which cause is the most common?
> Cardiac pump failure that causes reduced cardiac output
> Causes: MI (most common), cardiac contusion, valvular disease, cardiomyopathies

93. What is hypovolemic shock? What are some causes?
> Loss of intravascular volume

> Causes: Trauma, GI bleeding, vomiting, diarrhea, dehydration, burns

## *Hyperlipidemia*

94. What are the desirable levels of LDL? HDL? Total cholesterol? Triglycerides?

> LDL <100 mg/dL
> HDL >60 mg/dL
> Total cholesterol <200 mg/dL
> Triglycerides <150 mg/dL

95. What is the first line medication for hyperlipidemia?

> HMG-CoA reductase inhibitors (statins)

96. Which labs should be obtained and reviewed prior to starting a patient on a statin medication?

> Lipid Panel
> Liver Function Tests

97. What is the primary target in lipid lowering therapy to prevent coronary artery disease?

> Low density lipoprotein cholesterol (LDL-C)

98. What class of medication is the best for lowering triglycerides?

> Fibrates

99. What is the most effective class of drug to raise high density lipoprotein (HDL) cholesterol levels?

> Niacin

100. Omega 3 fatty acids can raise the level of which cholesterol?

> HDL

101. What are the most common adverse effects of statin therapy?

> ➤ Myalgia, limb pain, diarrhea, dyspepsia, arthralgia, elevated transaminases

102. What are two possible signs and symptoms of hypertriglyceridemia?

> ➤ Lipemia retinalis
> ➤ Pancreatitis

# Cardiomyopathy

## Dilated Cardiomyopathy

103. What is dilated cardiomyopathy?

> ➤ Dilation and impaired contraction of one or both ventricles
>   - Impaired systolic pump function which may lead to heart failure

104. What would you expect to see on an echocardiogram of a patient with dilated cardiomyopathy?

> ➤ LV dilation and reduced ejection fraction (EF)

105. What are some reversible causes of dilated cardiomyopathy?

> ➤ Alcohol abuse, pregnancy, thyroid disease, cocaine abuse, chronic uncontrolled tachycardia

106. What type of cardiomyopathy presents most commonly as chest pain in a woman after a stressful event?

> ➤ Takotsubo cardiomyopathy ("Broken Heart Syndrome")

107. In a patient with Takotsubo cardiomyopathy, what would you expect to see on EKG? On echocardiogram? What cardiac biomarkers may be

elevated? What findings would be present during cardiac catheterization?

> EKG – ST segment elevation
> Echocardiogram – regional wall motion abnormalities
> Cardiac biomarkers – possible troponin elevation
> Cardiac catheterization – apical ballooning in the absence of coronary artery disease (CAD)

## *Hypertrophic Cardiomyopathy*

108. What is the most common cause of sudden cardiac death in young athletes?

> Hypertrophic cardiomyopathy

109. What is the most common complaint patients have with hypertrophic cardiomyopathy?

> Dyspnea

110. What is the inheritance pattern for hypertrophic cardiomyopathy?

> Autosomal dominant (AD)

111. Hypertrophic cardiomyopathy is associated with what type of cardiac dysfunction?

> Diastolic

112. What are the characteristics of the murmur associated with hypertrophic cardiomyopathy? Where is it best heard?

> Mid-systolic, crescendo-decrescendo murmur
>   - Increases with decreased LV filling – Valsalva
>   - Decreases with increased LV filling – squatting
> Left lower sternal boarder

### *Restrictive Cardiomyopathy*

113. What is restrictive cardiomyopathy?
> ➢ Abnormal diastolic function
> ➢ Ventricular walls become stiff/rigid and impedes ventricular filling

114. What are the most common causes of restrictive cardiomyopathy?
> ➢ Idiopathic
> ➢ Amyloidosis
> ➢ Sarcoidosis
> ➢ Hemochromatosis
> ➢ Radiation

115. What symptoms are seen in a patient with restrictive cardiomyopathy?
> ➢ Right sided congestive heart failure (CHF)
> ➢ Kussmaul's sign – increase in jugular venous pressure (JVP) with inspiration

## Coronary Artery Disease

116. What are common risk factors for CAD and acute coronary syndrome (ACS)?
> ➢ Diabetes
> ➢ Hypertension
> ➢ Hyperlipidemia
> ➢ Family history
> ➢ Male gender
> ➢ Obesity
> ➢ Sedentary lifestyle
> ➢ Prior history of MI

> Smoking

117. What is the initial test used to determine the presence of CAD in a patient who is not actively having chest pain, acute EKG changes, or elevated biomarkers?

> Stress test (exercise or chemical)

118. What is the definition of stable angina?

> Substantial chest pain or discomfort aggravated by exercise and alleviated by rest or administration of nitroglycerin

119. What is the definition of unstable angina?

> Acute chest pain or discomfort while at rest

120. What is Prinzmetal's variant angina? What EKG finding is this associated with?

> Coronary artery vasospasm
> Ischemic pain that occurs at rest, not usually with exertion
> Transient ST-segment elevation

121. What is the main treatment for Prinzmetal's variant angina?

> Nitrates
> Calcium channel blockers

122. What study is the gold standard to evaluate obstructive coronary artery disease?

> Coronary angiography

123. What is NSTEMI? STEMI?

> NSTEMI – cardiac chest pain with elevation of troponin in the absence of ST elevation on EKG

> STEMI – cardiac chest pain with elevation of troponin in the presence of ST elevation on EKG

124. What are typical symptoms of an acute MI?

> Substernal chest pressure that radiates to the left arm or jaw, worsens with exertion
> - Often associated with diaphoresis, nausea, and vomiting

125. What patient populations are at an increased risk of presenting with nonclassical symptoms of an acute MI?

> Elderly, women, and diabetics

126. What is diagnostic of a STEMI on EKG?

> ST segment elevation >1 mm in 2 contiguous leads

127. What EKG leads correlate with each type of MI and what is the vessel that supplies that area?

> Septal – V1-V2
> - Left anterior descending (LAD)
> Anterior – V3-V4
> - Left anterior descending (LAD)
> Lateral – V5-V6, I, aVL
> - Left circumflex (LCx)
> Inferior – II, III, aVF
> - Right coronary artery (RCA)

128. What mnemonic is used to recall which leads show reciprocal changes in an MI?

> **PAILS**
> - **P**osterior MI → **A**nterior ST depression
> - **A**nterior MI → **I**nferior ST depression

- **I**nferior MI → **L**ateral ST depression
- **L**ateral MI → **S**eptal (and inferior) ST depression
- **S**eptal MI → **P**osterior ST depression

129. What cardiac biomarkers are elevated in the event of an acute MI?

> Myoglobin, troponin I, troponin T, CK-MB

130. Which cardiac biomarker is the most specific?

> Troponin

131. What is the HEART score?

> A risk stratification tool for ACS in patients who present with chest pain
> Components – **H**istory, **E**KG, **A**ge, **R**isk factors, **T**roponin

132. What is the treatment of ACS?

> **M**orphine, **O**xygen, **N**itroglycerine, **A**spirin, **B**eta blocker
- Remember: "**MONAB**"

133. What is the time goal for reperfusion in a patient with ACS?

> PCI within 90 minutes of first contact

134. In a non-PCI capable hospital that is >120 minutes away from the closest PCI center, what therapy should be administered for management of ST elevation myocardial infarction?

> Fibrinolytic

135. What medications are indicated for post myocardial infarction?

> Beta blockers, aspirin, P2Y12 inhibitor, high intensity statin, ACE inhibitor

136. What is Levine's sign?
> Patient holds a clenched fist over their chest when describing their chest pain

137. What is Dressler's Syndrome? What is the treatment?
> Pericarditis occurring 2-10 weeks following MI
> NSAIDS or corticosteroids

## *Valvular Disorders*

138. What are the systolic murmurs?
> Mitral Regurgitation
> Aortic Stenosis
> Pulmonic Stenosis
> Tricuspid Regurgitation

139. What are types of diastolic murmurs?
> Mitral Stenosis
> Aortic Regurgitation
> Pulmonic regurgitation
> Tricuspid Stenosis

140. What are the two types of valvular disorders?
> Stenosis – narrowing
> Insufficiency/regurgitation – retrograde blood flow

141. What is the best imaging modality for diagnosing valvular disorders?
> Echocardiogram

142. What is the most common valvular disorder?
> Aortic stenosis

143. Where is a murmur caused by aortic stenosis best heard? Mitral regurgitation? Pulmonary stenosis? Tricuspid insufficiency?

> Aortic stenosis: Right upper sternal border
> Mitral Regurgitation: Left 5th intercostal space, midclavicular line (apex)
> Pulmonary stenosis: Left upper sternal border
> Tricuspid insufficiency: Left lower sternal border

144. Where is a murmur caused by aortic regurgitation best heard? Mitral stenosis? Pulmonary insufficiency? Tricuspid stenosis?

> Aortic regurgitation: Left upper sternal border
  - Only murmur that does NOT match with its corresponding location
> Mitral stenosis: Left 5th intercostal space, midclavicular line (apex)
> Pulmonary insufficiency: Left upper sternal border
> Tricuspid stenosis: Left lower sternal border

145. What are the classic symptoms associated with severe aortic stenosis?

> Chest pain
> Syncope
> Dyspnea

146. What are the most common causes of aortic stenosis?

> Atherosclerosis
> Congenital (bicuspid valve)
> Rheumatic heart disease

147. How is the murmur for aortic stenosis described?

> Systolic murmur
> Harsh, crescendo-decrescendo sound

148. What medications are contraindicated in a patient with aortic stenosis?
> Nitrates, beta blockers, and calcium channel blockers

149. How do pulmonic and tricuspid valve disorders typically present?
> Right sided HF

# Conduction Disorders & Dysrhythmias

## _Atrial Fibrillation (AF)_

150. What is the most common cardiac arrhythmia?
> Atrial Fibrillation (AF)

151. What are the most common causes of AF?
> Hypertension
> Valvular disorders
> CAD
> Hyperthyroidism
> Alcohol use ("holiday heart")
> Idiopathic

152. How is AF classified?
> Paroxysmal: AF which terminates spontaneously or with intervention within 7 days of onset
> Persistent: Continuous AF that is sustained >7 days
> Long-standing persistent: Continuous AF >12 months

> Permanent: When the clinician and patient mutually decide that rhythm control will not be further attempted and the patient will remain in atrial fibrillation

153. What is AF with rapid ventricular response (RVR)?

> AF that elicits a ventricular response of >120 bpm

154. What EKG findings are seen with atrial fibrillation?

> No discernable P-waves
> Irregularly irregular rhythm

155. What hormone level should always be checked in a patient with newly diagnosed AF?

> Thyroid-stimulating hormone (TSH)

156. What are the two focuses of treatment for AF? What medication classes are used?

> Rate control – beta blockers or calcium channel blockers
> Rhythm control – synchronized cardioversion or chemical cardioversion

157. What is the treatment of an unstable patient with AF?

> Synchronized cardioversion

158. What are the two primary cardiovascular complications of AF?

> Cardiomyopathy and thromboembolism

159. What is the most common arterial thromboembolic complication of AF?

> Stroke

160. What is the drug of choice in patients with AF and valvular disease (ie. severe mitral stenosis, mechanical prosthetic valve)?

> Warfarin (coumadin)

161. What are the drugs of choice in patients with AF without valvular disease (non-valvular AF)?

> Direct-Acting Oral Anticoagulants (DOAC):
    Apixaban, rivaroxaban, dabigatran, edoxaban

162. What anticoagulant is used in patients with AF who have a mechanical heart valve?

> Warfarin
    - INR goal: 2.5-3.5

163. What is the antidote for Warfarin?

> Vitamin K

## Sinus Bradycardia

164. What are the common metabolic disorders that can cause sinus bradycardia?

> Sepsis, hypothermia, hypoxia, and hypoglycemia

## Heart Block

165. What are the types of AV blocks? What EKG characteristics are associated with each?

> First-degree
    - PR constantly prolonged
> Second-degree
    - Mobitz type I/Wenckebach – PR progressively lengthened with dropped beats
        - Remember: "Longer, longer longer, drop, now you've got Wenckebach"

- Mobitz type II – PR constantly prolonged with dropped beats
➢ Third-degree/complete heart block – complete AV dissociation

166. What are the treatment options for an AV block? Which require a pacemaker?
➢ Treatment – atropine, pacing
➢ Require pacemaker – second-degree Mobitz type II, third-degree/complete heart block

167. What is a characteristic EKG finding in a right bundle branch block?
➢ RSR' V1-V3 (rabbit ears)

168. A new left bundle branch block is suspicious for what pathology?
➢ Myocardial infarction (MI)

## Supraventricular Dysrhythmias

169. What is first line treatment in a stable patient with supraventricular tachycardia (SVT)? What medication can be used if its refractory?
➢ Vagal maneuvers
➢ Adenosine

170. What is first line treatment in an unstable patient with SVT?
➢ Synchronized cardioversion

171. What classic pulmonary disease is associated with multifocal atrial tachycardia?
➢ COPD

172. What is slurred upstroke of the QRS on an EKG called? What dysrhythmia is it associated with?

> Delta Wave
> Wolff-Parkinson-White (WPW)
>   ▪ Also referred to as paroxysmal supraventricular tachycardia

173. What is the abnormality found in Wolff-Parkinson-White Syndrome?
> Bundle of Kent accessory pathway which connects the atria to the ventricles

174. What is the definitive treatment in a patient with WPW?
> Catheter ablation

175. What is the condition that is caused by impairment or damage to the SA node?
> Sick Sinus Syndrome

## *Ventricular Dysrhythmias*

176. What is Torsades de Pointes (TdP)?
> Polymorphic ventricular tachycardia
>   ▪ QRS swings from positive to negative ("twisting of the points")

177. What is the treatment for TdP?
> IV magnesium sulfate
> If refractory and unstable with pulse – cardioversion
> If refractory, unstable and pulseless – defibrillation

178. What are the two shockable rhythms that require defibrillation?
> Pulseless ventricular tachycardia
> Ventricular fibrillation

179. What is ventricular tachycardia (VT) commonly associated with?
  ➤ Ischemic heart disease/MI

180. What EKG findings are seen in a patient with VT?
  ➤ Wide, fast rhythm (>100 bpm)

181. What is the treatment for VT in a stable patient? Unstable patient?
  ➤ Stable – antiarrhythmics (amiodarone, lidocaine, procainamide)
  ➤ Unstable
    ▪ Pulse – synchronized cardioversion
    ▪ Pulseless – defibrillation

182. What EKG findings are seen in a patient with VF?
  ➤ Zig-zag pattern with no P-waves, QRS complexes, or T-waves

183. What is the initial treatment for VF?
  ➤ Immediate defibrillation

## Heart Failure

184. What are the most common causes of left sided heart failure?
  ➤ Hypertension
  ➤ CAD/MI
  ➤ Cardiomyopathies
  ➤ Valvular heart disease
  ➤ Dysrhythmias

185. What is the most common cause of right sided heart failure? Symptoms?
  ➤ Cause – left sided heart failure

➢ Symptoms – peripheral edema, anorexia, nausea, fatigue

186. What are common symptoms of left sided heart failure?

➢ Dyspnea, cough, fatigue, orthopnea, paroxysmal nocturnal dyspnea (PND), exercise intolerance

187. What are the most common signs and symptoms of acute heart failure?

➢ Hypotension, pulmonary edema, cardiogenic shock

188. What are common physical exam findings for heart failure?

➢ Rales, rhonchi, tachycardia, peripheral edema, jugular venous distention (JVD), hepatojugular reflux (HJR)

189. What might you see on chest x-ray in a patient with decompensated heart failure?

➢ Kerley B lines
➢ Alveolar edema (bat wing appearance)
➢ Pulmonary congestion
➢ Cardiomegaly
➢ Pleural effusion

190. What is the test of choice to measure EF in heart failure?

➢ Echocardiogram

191. What is the difference between systolic and diastolic heart failure?

➢ Systolic heart failure – reduced EF (HFrEF); EF <40%

➢ Diastolic heart failure – preserved EF (HFpEF); EF >50%

192. What is the recommended fluid restriction and dietary sodium restrictions for patients with heart failure?

➢ Fluids: 1.5-2L/day
➢ Sodium restriction: 2-3 grams daily

193. What biomarkers are used to help diagnose patients with heart failure?

➢ B-type natriuretic peptide (BNP)
    ▪ N-terminal pro-BNP may also be used

194. What are Cheyne-Stokes respirations? In what condition are they common?

➢ Cyclic respiration in which the patient has periods of apnea followed by hyperpnea, decreased respiratory rate, and ultimately the next apneic period
➢ Advanced heart failure

195. What is another name for right sided heart failure?

➢ Cor Pulmonale

196. What medications are used for the chronic maintenance of heart failure?

➢ ACE/ARB
➢ Beta blocker
➢ Aldosterone receptor antagonist (spironolactone)
➢ Thiazide or loop diuretics (symptomatic treatment)

197. At what EF does a patient require an internal cardiac defibrillator (ICD)?

➢ ≤35%

# *Heart Inflammation*

## *Pericarditis*

198. What is acute pericarditis?
> ➢ Inflammation of the pericardial sac

199. What are the classic signs and symptoms of pericarditis?
> ➢ Pleuritic chest pain
> > ▪ Pain may be relieved by sitting up or leaning forward
> ➢ Pericardial friction rub
> > ▪ To-and-fro sound of the heart rubbing on the pericardium

200. What EKG findings are classically seen with pericarditis?
> ➢ Diffuse ST-segment elevations
> ➢ PR depression

201. What is the treatment for pericarditis?
> ➢ NSAIDs
> ➢ Colchicine

202. What is a Pericardial effusion?
> ➢ Accumulation of excess fluid within the pericardial sac

203. What are the physical exam findings in a patient with a pericardial effusion?
> ➢ Faint heart sounds
> ➢ Pericardial friction rub and apex impulse may disappear

> Ewart's sign (dullness on percussion near left
scapular region)

204. What is a chest x-ray finding seen with pericardial effusion?

> "Water Bottle" appearance to the cardiac silhouette

205. What is the treatment for recurrent pericardial effusions?

> Pericardial window

206. What is a potentially fatal complication of pericarditis?

> Cardiac tamponade

207. What are the three presenting features of cardiac tamponade, also known as Beck's Triad?

> Hypotension
> Soft or absent heart sounds
> Jugular venous distention (JVD)

208. What is pulsus paradoxus? In which conditions may this occur?

> Exaggerated drop in systolic blood pressure during inspiration
> Cardiac tamponade

209. What would you see on echocardiogram in a patient with cardiac tamponade?

> RA/RV collapse

210. What Is the treatment of cardiac tamponade?

> Pericardiocentesis

## *Endocarditis*

211. What is infective endocarditis?

> Infection of the endothelial lining of the heart
> Usually involving the heart valves

212. What are the most common risk factors for endocarditis?

> Valvular disease
> Prosthetic valve
> IV drug use

213. What is the most common pathogen seen with all types of infective endocarditis?

> Staphylococcus aureus

214. What are some physical findings of infective endocarditis?

> Fever
> Heart Murmur
  ▪ New or change to existing murmur
> Splenomegaly
> Janeway lesions
> Osler nodes
> Roth spots

215. What is the most common valve affected in endocarditis?

> Tricuspid

216. What highly sensitive and specific scoring tool is used to aid in the diagnosis of infective endocarditis?

> Duke Criteria

217. What diagnostic test is best for visualizing cardiac vegetations?

> Transesophageal echocardiography (TEE)

218. What is the treatment for endocarditis?

> Empiric antibiotics after 3 sets of blood cultures

219. What is the primary cause of death for patients with infective endocarditis?

> Congestive heart failure

220. What are Osler's nodes? Janeway lesions? Roth spots?

> Osler's nodes: Painful, violet-colored nodules on the fingers or toes

> Janeway lesions: Painless, red spots on the palms or soles

> Roth spots: White centered retinal hemorrhages

221. What are splinter hemorrhages? With what condition are they most commonly associated?

> Subungual, linear hemorrhages

> Infective endocarditis

## Congenital Heart Disease

222. What is the most common congenital heart disorder?

> Ventricular septal defect (VSD)

223. Which type of atrial septal defect is most common?

> Ostium secundum-type defect

224. What disorder is coarctation of the aorta (CoA) associated with?

> Turner Syndrome

225. What are some signs and symptoms of CoA?

> Hypertension (arms > legs)

> Brachial-femoral pulse delay

226. What is a patent ductus arteriosus (PDA)?

> Patency of the ductus arteriosus (structure that bypasses the pulmonary vasculature and connects the pulmonary artery to the aorta) that persists after birth

227. What is the most common cyanotic congenital heart defect?

> Tetralogy of Fallot

228. What are the main features of Tetralogy of Fallot?

> **P**ulmonic stenosis
> **R**ight Ventricular Hypertrophy (RVH)
> **O**verriding aorta
> **V**entricular Septal Defect
  - Remember: "**PROV**"

229. What is the classic symptom of Tetralogy of Fallot? What will the patient do to relieve symptoms?

> Tet spells – cyanosis with feeding or crying
> Squat down

230. What is the classic chest x-ray finding in a patient with Tetralogy of Fallot?

> Boot-shaped heart


## Vascular Diseases

### Aortic Aneurysms

231. What are the risk factors for aortic aneurysms?

> Male gender
> Increasing age
> Smoking
> Hypertension
> Family history

> Connective tissue disorders – Ehlers-Danlos, Marfan's syndrome

232. What is the most common predisposing factor for a dissecting aortic aneurysm?

> Hypertension

233. What findings may appear on chest x-ray in a patient with a dissecting aortic aneurysm?

> Widened mediastinum
> Tracheal deviation
> Double aortic knob
> Irregular aortic knob

234. What is the classic triad of symptoms in a ruptured abdominal aortic aneurysm?

> Abdominal pain
> Hypotension
> Pulsatile mass

235. What is the test of choice for diagnosing aortic dissections?

> CTA chest

236. What are the two systems used to classify aortic dissections?

> Stanford
> DeBakey

237. What is the difference between type A and type B dissections when using the Stanford classification?

> Type A: Dissection of ascending aorta
> Type B: Dissection of the descending aorta

238. What are the common presenting symptoms of an aortic dissection?

➢ Sudden, severe, tearing/ripping chest pain that
    radiates to the back, pulse deficits

239. What imaging modalities are used to evaluate for a
thoracic aortic aneurysm?

➢ CT and TTE/TEE

240. What imaging modalities are used to evaluate for
AAA?

➢ Abdominal ultrasound and CTA abdomen

241. What is first line medical therapy for acute aortic
dissection?

➢ IV beta blockers

242. What is the goal of blood pressure management
with acute aortic dissection?

➢ Rapidly lower systolic blood pressure
- Goal: 100 to 120 mmHg

## *Limb Ischemia*

243. What is acute limb ischemia?

➢ Sudden loss of blood flow to an extremity

244. What are the two main causes of an acute arterial
occlusion?

➢ Embolism
➢ Thrombus in situ

245. What is the most common risk factor for
developing acute limb ischemia from an embolic event?

➢ Atrial fibrillation

246. What is the classic presentation of limb ischemia?

➢ The 6 **P**s – **P**ain, **P**allor, **P**oikilothermia,
    **P**aresthesia, **P**ulselessness, **P**aralysis

247. What is the test of choice for diagnosing acute limb ischemia?
> CTA

248. What is the treatment for acute limb ischemia?
> Emergent surgical intervention

## *Peripheral Artery Disease (PAD)*

249. What is the clinical disorder that occurs when there is stenosis or an occlusion in the arteries of the limbs?
> Peripheral arterial disease (PAD)

250. What are the classic symptoms of PAD associated with intermittent claudication?
> Pain/aching in calves or buttock, relieves with rest

251. What are the common physical findings associated with PAD?
> Decreased or absent pulses, bruit over narrowed arteries, muscle atrophy, loss of hair, decreased skin temperature, shiny skin, pallor, ulcerations, gangrene

252. What ankle-brachial index (ABI) is considered diagnostic for peripheral arterial disease?
> < 0.90

253. What is the definitive treatment for PAD?
> Surgical/endovascular revascularization

## *Venous Thromboses*

254. What are the classic exam findings for superficial thromboses?

> Cordlike superficial vein
> Warm and tender to palpation
> Erythematous and edematous soft tissues

255. What are the most common causes of phlebitis/thrombophlebitis?

> IV or PICC lines

256. What is the treatment for superficial vein thrombosis?

> NSAIDs
> Warm compresses
> Elevation of extremity

## Deep Vein Thrombosis (DVT)

257. What is the typical presentation of a DVT?

> Unilateral leg swelling/pain, redness, and tenderness
> +/- positive Homan's sign – calf pain with dorsiflexion of the foot

258. What imaging is used to diagnosis a DVT?

> Doppler ultrasound

259. What other findings of leg pain may be identified on ultrasound if a DVT is not identified?

> Baker's Cyst
> Hematoma

260. Patients with a DVT are at risk for what potentially life-threatening complication?

> Pulmonary embolism

## *Chronic Venous Insufficiency*

261. What are common signs and symptoms of venous insufficiency?
   ➤ Dull/aching pain, pitting edema, varicose veins, brawny skin, ulceration (medial malleoli)
262. What is the treatment for venous insufficiency?
   ➤ Graduated compression stockings, elevation
263. What is Virchow's triad?
   ➤ Stasis, endothelial injury, and hypercoagulability

# Cardiovascular System

# 3

---

# PULMONARY SYSTEM

## *General Pulmonology*

264. What are the four measurements of lung volumes?
   ➢ Tidal volume (TV): Air that enters the lungs with each normal effort inspiration
   ➢ Residual volume (RV): Air remaining in lung after maximal expiration
   ➢ Expiratory reserve volume (ERV): Air that can be further exhaled after normal tidal volume expiration
   ➢ Inspiratory reserve volume (IRV): Air that can be inhaled after normal tidal volume inspiration

265. What are the four capacities measured in the lung?
   ➢ Inspiratory capacity = IRV + TV
   ➢ Functional residual capacity = RV + ERV
   ➢ Vital capacity = TV + IRV + ERV
   ➢ Total lung capacity = IRV + TV + ERV + RV

266. What are the three categories for the duration of a cough?
   ➢ Acute: <3 weeks
   ➢ Subacute: Between 3 to 8 weeks
   ➢ Chronic: >8 weeks

267. What are the three most common causes of chronic cough in a patient who is a nonsmoker with a normal chest x-ray and not taking any medications?
   ➢ Postnasal drip or upper airway cough syndrome
   ➢ Asthma
   ➢ GERD

268. When inspiratory stridor is auscultated, what type of airway disease is this indicative of?
   ➢ Upper Airway Disease

269. What type of airway disease are expiratory wheezes or rhonchi indicative of?

> Lower Airway Disease

270. Inspiratory crackles are most commonly heard with what three lung processes?

> Pneumonia
> Pulmonary edema
> Interstitial lung disease

271. What blood pressure medication may cause a chronic cough?

> ACE inhibitors

272. What is the procedure of choice in assessing an endobronchial tumor?

> Fiberoptic bronchoscopy
> ▪ May also obtain cytologic and histologic specimens during this procedure

273. What are some contraindications for noninvasive positive pressure ventilation (NIPPV)?

> Altered mental status
> Copious secretions/unable to clear secretions
> Poor fitting of the mask
> ▪ Craniofacial abnormalities
> ▪ Trauma
> Extreme obesity
> Significant burns
> Cardiovascular instability

274. What are some contraindications for beta blocker medications?

> Asthma, COPD, emphysema, chronic
  bronchitis, sinus bradycardia, second degree heart
  block, third degree heart block

275. What are the common signs of respiratory distress
in infants and children?

> Tachypnea, retractions, nasal flaring, accessory
  muscle use, grunting, wheezing, stridor, sweating,
  color change to mouth/lips/fingernails

276. What results are seen in pulmonary function
testing with restrictive lung disease? Obstructive lung
disease?

> Restrictive
  - FEV1/FVC: Normal/increased
  - TLC: Decreased
> Obstructive
  - FEV1/FVC: Decreased
  - TLC: Increased

277. What is the most common location for an
aspirated foreign body?

> Right mainstem bronchus

## Pulmonary Infections

### Pneumonia

278. What are the two main categories of pneumonia?

> Community acquired pneumonia (CAP)
> Hospital-acquired pneumonia (HAP)
  - Includes ventilator associated pneumonia
    (VAP)

279. What are the most common causes of typical pneumonia?

> S. pneumoniae, H. influenzae, Klebsiella, S. aureus, Pseudomonas

280. What are the most common causes of atypical pneumonia?

> Mycoplasma pneumoniae, Chlamydia pneumoniae, Legionella, Chlamydia psittaci, viruses

281. What screening tools are used to determine disposition of patients with pneumonia?

> Pneumonia severity index
> **CURB-65**
  - **C**onfusion
  - **U**remia
  - **R**espiratory rate
  - **B**lood pressure
  - Age >**65**

282. What would you see on chest x-ray in a patient with pneumonia?

> Typical – lobar consolidation
> Atypical – diffuse consolidation

283. What is the most common cause of a lung abscess?

> Aspiration pneumonia

284. What etiology of pneumonia must be considered in a patient with HIV and a CD4 count <200?

> Pneumocystis jirovecii (formerly known as PCP)

285. What are patients with viral pneumonia at risk for?

> Secondary bacterial infection

## *Tuberculosis*

286. What are some immunologic and environmental risk factors for developing tuberculosis?

> ➤ Impaired immunity: HIV, DM, immunosuppressant medications, transplant patients, substance abuse, malnutrition, malignancy, renal disease, gastric surgery, celiac disease, cirrhosis, COPD
> ➤ Environmental factors: Household contact, birth in a TB-endemic region, hospitals, correctional facilities, nursing homes, homeless shelters, low socioeconomic status, minorities

287. What are some common symptoms of tuberculosis?

> ➤ Fever, night sweats, cough, hemoptysis, weight loss, fatigue

288. What is the screening test for tuberculosis?

> ➤ PPD skin test or Interferon Gamma Release Assay (IGRA) blood test

289. If a patient has a positive TB test (ie. PPD), what is the next diagnostic test that should be performed?

> ➤ Chest x-ray

290. What are the classic x-ray findings associated with tuberculosis?

> ➤ Cavitation
> ➤ Upper lope infiltrates
> ➤ Hilar/paratracheal lymphadenopathy
> ➤ Ghon complexes
> ➤ Ranke complexes

291. How is the definitive diagnosis of tuberculosis made?
> Positive Mycobacterium tuberculosis sputum culture

292. What is the treatment for tuberculosis? What side effects are seen with each medication?
> "**RIPE**" therapy for 6-9 months
  - **R**ifampin – orange bodily fluids
  - **I**soniazid – vitamin B6 deficiency
  - **P**yrazinamide – hepatotoxicity
  - **E**thambutol – optic neuritis

## *Bronchiolitis*

293. What is the most common cause of acute bronchiolitis?
> Respiratory Syncytial Virus (RSV)

294. How does acute bronchiolitis typically present?
> Cough, nasal congestion, wheezing, coarse breath sounds

295. What is the treatment for acute bronchiolitis?
> Supportive care (unless severely ill, premature, apneic, immunocompromised)
  - Nasal suctioning
  - Humidified $O_2$

## *Bronchitis*

296. What is the most common cause of acute bronchitis?
> Viral (adenovirus, rhinovirus)

297. What is the primary symptom of acute bronchitis?

> Cough +/- sputum

298. What is the primary treatment for bronchitis?
> Supportive care
- Antibiotics are not routinely recommended

## Croup

299. What is another name for croup? What is the most common cause?
> Acute laryngotracheobronchitis
> Parainfluenza virus

300. What is the most common age range for croup?
> 6 months to 6 years

301. How would a patient with croup present?
> Barky seal-like cough, inspiratory stridor, increased work of breathing

302. What classically improves the symptoms of croup?
> Cool night air

303. What is the classic x-ray finding in croup?
> Steeple sign

304. If a patient with croup has stridor at rest, what medication should be given?
> Racemic epinephrine

## Epiglottitis

305. What are the three classic symptoms for epiglottitis?
> Abrupt onset of fever, stridor, respiratory distress
- Tripod positioning, sore throat, drooling, anxiety, dysphagia may also be present

306. What imaging is helpful for diagnosing epiglottitis?
> Soft tissue lateral neck xray

307. What is the classic sign seen on x-ray in epiglottitis?
> Thumb sign
  - Caused by an edematous and enlarged epiglottis

308. Which immunization has decreased the incidence of epiglottitis infections? When is the vaccine administered?
> Haemophilus influenzae type B vaccination (Hib vaccine)
> Given at age 2 months and 4 months (two dose series) or age 2, 4, and 6 months (three dose series) depending on formulation
  - Booster dose at 12-15 months old

309. What are now the leading pathogens of epiglottitis since era of the Hib vaccine?
> Streptococcus
> Staphylococcus

310. What is the initial treatment for acute epiglottitis?
> Secure airway first, then IV antibiotics

## Influenza

311. What are the peak months for influenza?
> December through March

312. What are the signs and symptoms of influenza?
> Fever, chills, rigors, dry cough, myalgias, malaise, headache, fatigue

313. What populations are at highest risk for serious influenza complications?
> Extreme ages (<6 months and >65 years old)
> Pregnant women
> Immunocompromised
> Residents of nursing homes/long-term care facilities
> Morbidly obese

314. Which patients should be given Oseltamivir for influenza?
> Symptomatic within 48 hours of symptom onset
> High-risk patients

## Pertussis

315. What is another name for pertussis?
> Whooping cough

316. What are the three stages of pertussis infection?
> Catarrhal – nonspecific symptoms
> Paroxysmal – paroxysms of coughing with inspiratory whoop, post-tussive vomiting
> Convalescent – gradual resolution of symptoms

317. At what age does the CDC recommend a child's first pertussis vaccination be given?
> 2 months old (DTaP vaccine)

318. When should infants and children be hospitalized for pertussis infection?
> Respiratory distress, evidence of pneumonia, cyanosis, apnea, seizures, <4 months old, inability to feed

## *Obstructive Airway Disease*

### COPD

319. What is a major risk factor for mortality from chronic bronchitis and emphysema?

> ➢ Cigarette smoking

320. What are the three most common symptoms of COPD?

> ➢ Cough
> ➢ Sputum production
> ➢ Exertional dyspnea

321. What are common signs and symptoms of chronic bronchitis?

> ➢ "Blue bloaters" – productive cough, dyspnea, peripheral edema, cyanosis, rales, wheezing

322. What are common signs and symptoms of chronic emphysema?

> ➢ "Pink puffers" – dyspnea on exertion, pursed-lip breathing, weight loss, increased AP diameter/barrel chest, quiet lungs

323. What are the classic chest x-ray findings for COPD?

> ➢ Increased lung markings (ie. chronic bronchitis)
> ➢ Hyperinflated lungs, flattened diaphragms, bullae/blebs (ie. chronic emphysema)

324. In COPD, what is the hallmark finding on PFTs?

> ➢ A decreased FEV1/FVC ratio of <0.7

325. What are the indications for continuous long-term oxygen therapy for patients with COPD?

> ➢ PaO2 ≤55 mmHg
> ➢ SpO2 ≤88% on room air at rest

326. What is the treatment for an acute COPD exacerbation?

> Short-acting muscarinic antagonist (SAMA)
> Short-acting beta agonist (SABA)
> Corticosteroids
> Supplemental $O_2$/NIPPV

327. What medications are used in the long-term management of COPD?

> Long-acting beta agonist (LABA)
> Long-acting muscarinic antagonist (LAMA)

328. What is Hoover's sign?

> Paradoxical inward movement of the rib cage with inspiration
  - May be seen in patients with advanced COPD

329. What are the 3 cardinal features of a COPD exacerbation?

> Increase in frequency of severity of cough
> Increase in sputum production or change in caliber
> Increased dyspnea

330. When are antibiotics indicated in COPD? Which antibiotics are commonly used?

> Severe exacerbations with change in sputum
> Azithromycin, 3rd generation cephalosporin, or doxycycline

331. What bacteria are frequently associated with COPD exacerbations?

> Streptococcus pneumoniae
> Haemophilus influenzae
> Moraxella catarrhalis

332. In a patient with COPD, what does an elevated hematocrit and signs of right ventricular hypertrophy suggest?

> Chronic hypoxemia

333. How is hypercarbia defined?

> Pco2 > 45mmHg

334. When should an arterial blood gas (ABG) be obtained in a patient with a COPD exacerbation?

> Advanced COPD patients
> History of hypercarbia
> Mental status change (ie. confusion, sleepiness)
> Significant respiratory distress

## _Asthma_

335. What is the gold standard for asthma diagnosis?

> Methacholine challenge

336. What is the atopic triad?

> Asthma, eczema, allergic rhinitis

337. What are common triggers for asthma exacerbations?

> Environmental/allergens
> Exercise
> Chemical irritants
> Upper respiratory infection (URI)

338. What test can be done in the office, or even at home, and be compared to prior values, to inform you of the severity of an asthma exacerbation?

> Peak flow meter

339. What are the asthma classifications? What are they based upon?

> Intermittent, mild persistent, moderate persistent, and severe persistent
> Symptom frequency, nighttime awakenings, use of SABA for symptoms, interference with activity, and lung function

340. What are the mainstays of treatment for long-term management of asthma?

> Stepwise approach
  - SABA PRN
  - Low, medium, or high-dose ICS
  - LABA
  - Oral Corticosteroids

341. What is the treatment for a mild/moderate asthma exacerbation?

> SABA/SAMA
> Corticosteroids

342. What are the main treatment options for severe asthma exacerbations that require admission?

> Albuterol nebulizer
> IV magnesium
> Systemic steroids
> Possible ventilatory support

343. What is the recommended treatment for occasional, exercise induced asthma?

> SABA 15-30 minutes before exercise

## *Restrictive Lung Disease*
### *Cystic Fibrosis*

344. What is the inheritance pattern of cystic fibrosis (CF)?
> ➤ Autosomal recessive

345. What organs does CF affect?
> ➤ Lungs, pancreas, liver, sinuses, sweat glands

346. What are the common symptoms of CF?
> ➤ Cough, recurrent pulmonary infections, failure to thrive, meconium ileus, pancreatitis

347. What is the test of choice for diagnosing CF?
> ➤ Sweat chloride test – >60 mEq/L on 2 occasions

348. What is a common chest x-ray finding seen in a patient with CF?
> ➤ Mucus plugging

### *Sarcoidosis*

349. What is sarcoidosis?
> ➤ Multisystem, inflammatory, granulomatous disease of unknown etiology

350. When does sarcoidosis typically present? What are the most common presenting symptoms of sarcoidosis?
> ➤ Primarily affects young and middle-aged adults
> ➤ Cough, dyspnea, chest pain
> ➤ May have eye lesions and/or skin lesions

351. What chest x-ray finding is commonly seen in sarcoidosis?

> Hilar lymphadenopathy

352. How is the definitive diagnosis of sarcoidosis made? What is the treatment?

> Biopsy: Non-caseating granulomas
> Treatment: Corticosteroids

## Idiopathic Pulmonary Fibrosis

353. What are some symptoms and physical exam findings of idiopathic pulmonary fibrosis?

> Exertional dyspnea, nonproductive cough, inspiratory crackles, digital clubbing

354. What is seen on chest x-ray and CT chest in a patient with idiopathic pulmonary fibrosis?

> Honeycombing

# Pleural Disease

## General

355. Where is the pleural space located?

> Between the lung and chest wall

356. What is a pleural effusion?

> Presence of excess fluid within the pleural space

357. What is an empyema?

> Infection within the pleural space

358. What is a hemothorax?

> The accumulation of blood within the pleural space

359. What is a pneumothorax?

> Presence of gas in the pleural space

## *Pleural Effusion*

360. What physical exam findings are associated with pleural effusions?

> ➤ Diminished lower lung sounds, dullness to percussion, decreased tactile fremitus

361. What would you see on x-ray in a patient with a pleural effusion?

> ➤ Blunting of the costophrenic angles

362. Small pleural effusions are best seen on which x-ray view?

> ➤ Lateral decubitus

363. What is the difference between a transudative and exudative pleural effusions? What are some common causes of each?

> ➤ Transudative – due to changes in hydrostatic/oncotic pressure, capillaries intact
>   - CHF, atelectasis, renal/liver disease
> ➤ Exudative – leaky capillaries
>   - Malignancy, infection, trauma

364. What is the diagnostic and therapeutic procedure performed for pleural effusions?

> ➤ Thoracentesis

365. What two levels are measured from the pleural fluid to differentiate between exudative and transudative pleural effusions?

> ➤ Lactate dehydrogenase (LDH)
> ➤ Protein levels

366. What are Lights Criteria?

> ➤ Pleural fluid protein >0.5 serum protein
> ➤ Pleural fluid LDH >0.6 serum LDH

> Pleural fluid LDH >2/3 upper limits of the laboratory reference range of serum LDH
> If any of the above 3 are positive, it is suggestive of an exudative effusion

367. What is the treatment for a complicated pleural effusion?
> Antibiotics
> Chest tube (they are at high risk for developing empyema)

368. What is the two leading causes for transudative pleural effusion in the United States?
> Left ventricular failure
> Cirrhosis

369. What are the leading causes for exudative pleural effusions?
> Bacterial pneumonia
> Malignancy
> Viral infection
> Pulmonary embolism

## Pneumothorax

370. What are some common physical exam findings seen with pneumothorax?
> Diminished breath sounds, hyperresonance to percussion, decreased tactile fremitus

371. What would be seen on x-ray in a patient with a pneumothorax?
> Absent lung markings
> Pleural-visceral line

372. What is the treatment for a pneumothorax?

➢ Small – supplemental $O_2$, observe, repeat x-ray

➢ Large or symptomatic – supplemental $O_2$, chest tube

373. What are some common physical exam findings seen in patient with a tension pneumothorax?

➢ JVD, hypotension, hypoxia, tachycardia, tracheal deviation (toward contralateral side)

374. How is tension pneumothorax treated?

➢ Large-bore needle decompression followed by a chest tube

375. Where should a chest tube be inserted?

➢ Fifth intercostal space at the midaxillary line

➢ Superior aspect of the rib to avoid the vein, artery, and nerve

376. Where is the preferred site for needle decompression of a pneumothorax?

➢ 2nd intercostal space midclavicular line

➢ Above the 3rd rib

377. What is the most common cause of secondary pneumothorax?

➢ Emphysema

## Pulmonary Circulation

### Pulmonary Embolism

378. What are the common signs and symptoms of a pulmonary embolism (PE)?

➢ Shortness of breath, pleuritic chest pain, hemoptysis, evidence of lower extremity DVT, tachycardia, tachypnea, hypoxia

379. What are the risk factors associated with pulmonary embolism?
  ➢ Prior PE or DVT, recent surgery, immobilization, active cancer, obesity, heavy smoker, oral contraception use, testosterone supplementation

380. What is the classic EKG finding seen with PE?
  ➢ S1Q3T3

381. What is the **PERC** rule for PE and how is it used?
  ➢ **P**ulmonary **E**mbolism **R**ule out **C**riteria – if any affirmative answer, PE <u>cannot</u> be ruled out
    ▪ >50-years-old
    ▪ Oxygen saturation <95%
    ▪ HR >100 bpm
    ▪ Unilateral leg swelling
    ▪ Hemoptysis
    ▪ Recent hospitalization or surgery within 4 weeks
    ▪ Prior history of DVT/PE
    ▪ Hormone use

382. What are the Well's Criteria for PE?
  ➢ Signs/symptoms of DVT (+3)
  ➢ PE is the most likely or equally likely diagnosis (+3)
  ➢ HR >100 (+1.5)
  ➢ Immobilization at least 3 days or surgery in the last 4 weeks (+1.5)
  ➢ Prior history of DVT/PE (+1.5)
  ➢ Hemoptysis (+1)
  ➢ Malignancy (+1)

383. What are the testing modalities for PE?
> Low risk (<2) – PERC rule
> Moderate risk (2-6) – D-dimer
> High risk (>6) – CT pulmonary angiography

384. What is the principal imaging test used for diagnosis of PE?
> CT angiogram of chest with IV contrast

385. What are the usual symptoms associated with massive PE versus small embolisms?
> Massive PE: Dyspnea, syncope, hypotension, cyanosis
> Small: Pleuritic chest pain, cough, hemoptysis

386. What are the treatment options for PE?
> Anticoagulation – heparin, LMWH, warfarin
> Thrombolysis/embolectomy

387. What is an option for prevention of PE recurrence in a patient who cannot tolerate anticoagulants?
> Inferior vena cava (IVC) filter

388. What are some methods used for PE prevention?
> Early ambulation
> SCDs
> Prophylactic anticoagulation – LMWH

389. What are two ways to assess for right ventricle heart strain secondary to PE? What would you expect to see?
> Transthoracic echocardiography
  ▪ Dilated right ventricle or hypokinesis of right ventricle wall
> Biomarkers: Elevated troponin levels, elevated BNP

390. What term is used to describe a large embolism that covers the bifurcation of the pulmonary trunk?
  ➤ Saddle pulmonary embolism

391. What is the most common cause of death from a PE?
  ➤ Progressive right heart failure

## *Pulmonary Hypertension*

392. What are the two most common presenting symptoms of patients with pulmonary hypertension?
  ➤ Exertional dyspnea
  ➤ Fatigue

393. As pulmonary hypertension progresses, what type of signs and symptoms develop?
  ➤ Right sided CHF

394. What is the initial test of choice when pulmonary hypertension is suspected?
  ➤ Transthoracic echocardiography (TTE)

395. What are the common etiologies for pulmonary hypertension?
  ➤ Pulmonary arterial hypertension
  ➤ Left sided heart disease
  ➤ Lung disease/hypoxia
  ➤ Thromboembolic disease
  ➤ Multifactorial

396. What would a right heart catheterization show in a patient with pulmonary hypertension?
  ➤ Mean pulmonary arterial pressure >20 mmHg at rest or >30 mmHg with exercise

397. What are some treatments used in the management of pulmonary hypertension?
> Treat the underlying disorder
> Anticoagulation
> Supplemental $O_2$
> Calcium channel blocker, prostacyclin

## Cor Pulmonale

398. What is cor pulmonale?
> Abnormal structure and function of the RV due to pulmonary hypertension
399. What are some common causes of cor pulmonale?
> COPD
> Pulmonary embolism
400. What would an echocardiogram show in patient with cor pulmonale?
> RVH and dilation of the RA

# Neoplasms

401. What are the most common types of lung cancer? Where are they most commonly located?
> Small-cell lung cancer (SCLC) – central
> Non-small-cell lung cancer
  ▪ Adenocarcinoma – peripheral
  ▪ Squamous cell carcinoma (SCC) – central
  ▪ Large cell carcinoma
402. What are common symptoms of lung cancer?
> Cough, hemoptysis, anorexia, weight loss

403. What electrolyte disturbance would you see in
SCLC?
  ➢ Hypercalcemia

404. How are lung cancers diagnosed?
  ➢ Biopsy
    ▪ Bronchoscopy – centrally located
    ▪ Transthoracic needle – peripherally located

405. What is the diagnostic test used in lung cancer
screening?
  ➢ Low dose CT

406. What are some characteristics of benign vs.
malignant pulmonary nodules?
  ➢ Benign – well-defined margins, slow growing,
    calcification
  ➢ Malignant – indistinct margins, spiculated,
    rapidly growing

## Sleep Apnea

407. What are some common disorders associated with
obstructive sleep apnea (OSA)?
  ➢ Obesity
  ➢ Hypertension
  ➢ Alcohol use

408. What are common symptoms of OSA?
  ➢ Hypersomnolence, snoring, decreased sexual
    desire, depression

409. What is the best test for evaluating for OSA?
  ➢ Polysomnography

410. What is the treatment for OSA?
  ➢ Lifestyle modifications/weight loss

> Continuous positive airway pressure (CPAP)

411. Untreated OSA can lead to what complications?

> Hypertension

> Pulmonary hypertension

## ARDS

412. What is acute respiratory distress syndrome (ARDS)? What are some common causes?

> An acute inflammatory reaction that results in non-cardiogenic pulmonary edema

> Sepsis, pneumonia, trauma, burns

413. What are the common signs and symptoms associated with ARDS?

> Sudden onset dyspnea, cough, severe hypoxemia refractory to supplemental $O_2$

414. What is the treatment for ARDS?

> Supportive care – ventilatory support

415. What other intervention in ARDS has been shown to reduce mortality in some studies?

> Prone positioning, lung protective mechanical ventilation

# Pulmonary System

# 4

---

# GASTROINTESTINAL
SYSTEM

## *General Gastroenterology*

416. What is the pathway food takes through the digestive system?

> Mouth → Esophagus → Stomach → Small Intestines (Duodenum → Jejunum → Ileum) → Colon → Cecum → Rectum → Anus

417. What is the most common abdominal surgical emergency?

> Appendicitis

418. What are peritoneal signs?

> Rebound tenderness
> Involuntary guarding

419. What does free air under the diaphragm on a plain abdominal x-ray indicated?

> Perforated viscus

420. What is an MRCP?

> Magnetic resonance cholangiopancreatography
> Noninvasive study used to visualize the biliary and pancreatic ducts

421. What is an ERCP?

> Endoscopic retrograde cholangiopancreatography
> Procedure using endoscopy and x-ray that diagnosis and treats a variety of pancreaticobiliary disorders including removal of stones in the bile ducts

422. What is the treatment for fecal impaction?

> Manual disimpaction, enema

423. What is the most common metabolic cause of gastroparesis?

➤ Diabetes mellitus

424. What promotility pharmacologic therapy is approved by the FDA for the management of gastroparesis?

> ➤ Metoclopramide

# *Small Intestine Disorders*

## *Celiac Disease*

425. What signs and symptoms should prompt testing for celiac disease?

> ➤ Signs of malabsorption such as diarrhea, weight loss, steatorrhea, bloating, postprandial abdominal pain, or findings such as early osteoporosis and iron-deficiency anemia

426. What lab marker is positive in celiac disease?

> ➤ Anti-tTG

427. What diet should patients with celiac disease adhere to?

> ➤ Gluten-free diet

## *Appendicitis*

428. What are the most common symptoms of appendicitis?

> ➤ Periumbilical pain, RLQ pain that is worse with movement, fever, chills, anorexia, nausea, vomiting, constipation

429. Where is McBurney's point? What is tenderness at this location suggestive of?

> ➤ 1/3 the distance from the ASIS to the umbilicus

➢ Appendicitis

430. What are other physical exam signs associated with appendicitis?

➢ Obturator Sign: Pain with internal rotation of the right hip

➢ Psoas Sign: Pain with extension of right hip

➢ Rovsing's Sign: Palpation to LLQ increases pain to RLQ

➢ Markle Sign: Dropping from standing on toes to heels or pounding lightly with closed fist on the patient's right heel produces RLQ pain

▪ Also called Heel Jar Test

431. What is the scoring tool that can be used to aid in the diagnosis of acute appendicitis?

➢ Modified Alvarado Score

432. What is an appendicolith? Can this cause appendicitis? How?

➢ Hard, calcified fecal matter

➢ Yes, may obstruct the appendix lumen resulting in appendicitis

▪ Most commonly an incidental finding on CT

433. What laboratory findings are typically seen with appendicitis?

➢ Leukocytosis with a left shift

▪ >10,000 WBC concern for acute appendicitis

▪ >20,000 WBC concern for perforated appendix

434. What does "left shift" mean?

➢ Increase in total WBC, neutrophils, & bands (immature neutrophils)

435. What is the treatment for appendicitis?
> Appendectomy +/- antibiotics

## *Intussusception*

436. What is the most common cause of intestinal obstruction in children between the ages of 6 months and 3 years old?
> Intussusception

437. What is intussusception?
> Telescoping of intestines into itself

438. How does intussusception present?
> Colicky abdominal pain, vomiting, currant jelly stool, sausage shaped mass, obstipation

439. What is the imaging modality of choice to diagnose intussusception?
> Ultrasound, CT

440. What is the non-surgical option for reduction of intussusception? When can this option be used?
> Air or oral contrast enema
> Clinically stable patients without signs of perforation, peritonitis, or shock

## *Small Bowel Obstruction (SBO)*

441. What are the most common causes of small bowel obstruction (SBO)?
> Adhesions (most common in patients with prior surgery)
> Tumors
> Hernias

442. How would a patient with bowel obstruction present?

> Colicky abdominal pain, distention, nausea, vomiting, constipation, incontinence of small amounts of liquid stool, PO intolerance

443. What would you hear on auscultation of a patient with bowel obstruction?

> Hyperactive high-pitched bowel sounds, hypoactive/absent bowel sounds

444. What would you see on abdominal x-ray in a patient with bowel obstruction?

> Multiple dilated loops of bowel
> Air-fluid levels

445. What is the best diagnostic test to evaluate for bowel obstruction?

> CT abdomen/pelvis with contrast

446. What is the treatment for bowel obstruction?

> NPO
> IV fluids
> Electrolyte repletion
> NG tube decompression
> Possible surgical intervention

## *Volvulus*

447. What is a volvulus? Where does it most commonly occur?

> Twisting of loops of bowel
> Sigmoid or cecum

## *Ileus*

448. What is an ileus? What are some common causes?
> Intestinal paralysis and bowel distention due to decreased or absent GI motility without an identifiable obstruction
> Post-op, electrolyte abnormalities

# *Biliary Disorders*

## *Cholecystitis*

449. What is cholelithiasis? What are common risk factors?
> Presence of gallstones in the gallbladder
> Female gender, obesity, child-bearing age, family history

450. How does cholelithiasis present?
> Most commonly asymptomatic
> Possible biliary colic – postprandial RUQ or epigastric abdominal pain, nausea

451. What is acute cholecystitis? What is the most common cause?
> Inflammation of the gallbladder secondary to obstruction of the cystic duct
> Infectious - infection caused by bacterial overgrowth secondary to gallbladder distention/biliary stasis from obstruction of the cystic duct
  - Most common bacteria - gram-negative bacteria, Escherichia coli

> Cholelithiasis (gallstones) is the most common cause

452. What is acalculous cholecystitis? In what patient populations might this be seen?

> Inflammation of the gallbladder without gallstones or sludge

> ICU, post-op, prolonged fasting, TPN, dehydration

453. How does acute cholecystitis present?

> Colicky RUQ pain that becomes constant, +/- nausea/vomiting, anorexia, fever

> Commonly after a high-fat meal

454. What is Murphy's sign?

> The examiner asks the patient to breathe in and then firmly palpates the RUQ

> Positive test – cessation of inspiration secondary to pain (suggestive of acute cholecystitis)

455. What imaging modality best visualizes the gallbladder? What are common findings in acute cholecystitis?

> RUQ ultrasound

> +/- Gallstones or sludge, gallbladder wall thickening (>4 mm), pericholecystic fluid, sonographic Murphy's sign

456. What is the confirmatory test for acute cholecystitis?

> HIDA scan (often not necessary to perform)

457. What is the definitive treatment for acute cholecystitis?

> Cholecystectomy

458. What is choledocholithiasis?
> The presence of one or more gallstones within the common bile duct

459. What are the two major complications associated with choledocholithiasis?
> Acute pancreatitis
> Acute cholangitis

460. What is cholangitis?
> Ascending infection of the biliary tree due to common bile duct obstruction (choledocholithiasis)

## Colorectal Disorders

### Diverticulosis

461. What are the most common areas affected by diverticular disease?
> Sigmoid and descending colon

462. What is the difference between diverticulosis and diverticulitis? How do they typically present?
> Diverticulosis – increased intraluminal pressure leading to mucosal outpouching between the taneia where the vasa recta enter the colonic wall
  ▪ Painless rectal bleeding
> Diverticulitis – inflammation/infection of diverticula
  ▪ Fever, change in bowel habits (diarrhea or constipation), constant LLQ pain, nausea, vomiting

463. What is the best test to evaluate for diverticulitis if complicated or no response to treatment?

➢ CT abdomen/pelvis

464. What diagnostic test is contraindicated during an acute bout of diverticulitis but is recommended after resolution of symptoms to rule out malignancy?

➢ Colonoscopy in 6 weeks post resolution of acute infection

465. What are the treatments for uncomplicated and complicated diverticulitis?

➢ Uncomplicated: PO antibiotics
➢ Complicated: IV antibiotics, NPO, possible surgical intervention

466. What are complications that occur with diverticulitis that typical require hospitalization and/or surgery?

➢ Frank perforation
➢ Obstruction
➢ Fistula
➢ Abscess


## Inflammatory Bowel Disease (IBD)

467. What are the two major types of IBD?

➢ Crohn's disease
➢ Ulcerative colitis

468. What is the typical age onset of ulcerative colitis and Crohn's disease?

➢ 15-30 years old with another peak at 50-70 years old

469. What is the diagnostic tool used to diagnose IBD?

➢ Colonoscopy with biopsy (not during an acute flare)

➢ UGI with small bowel follow through for
  Crohn's disease

470. Which IBD primarily causes fistula formation and
anal disease to occur?

➢ Crohn's disease

471. What is the treatment for an acute flare of IBD?

➢ IV fluids
➢ High-dose corticosteroids
➢ Antibiotics

472. What malignancy does IBD increase a patient's
risk for?

➢ Colorectal cancer

473. Where does abdominal pain most commonly
present in patients with Crohn's disease? Ulcerative
Colitis?

➢ Crohn's disease: Right lower quadrant abdomen
➢ Ulcerative colitis: Left lower quadrant abdomen

474. What locations of the GI tract are affected by
Crohn's disease? Ulcerative colitis?

➢ Crohn's disease: Mouth to anus
➢ Ulcerative colitis: Colon/rectum

475. Which IBD may occur with arthralgia and
arthritis?

➢ Ulcerative colitis

476. What are some associated skin manifestations seen
with IBD?

➢ Erythema nodosum
➢ Pyoderma gangrenosum
➢ Skin tags

477. How does a patient with Crohn's disease present?

➢ Fever, crampy abdominal pain (most commonly RLQ), diarrhea, fatigue, weight loss

478. What are the most common signs and symptoms seen in patients with ulcerative colitis?

➢ Bloody diarrhea (hallmark)
➢ Rectal bleeding
➢ Passage of mucus
➢ Abdominal pain (most common LLQ)
➢ Tenesmus
➢ Proctitis

479. What is tenesmus?

➢ Sensation for the need to pass stool, even after having a bowel movement

480. Is ulcerative colitis or Crohn's disease more closely linked with toxic megacolon?

➢ Ulcerative colitis

481. What is toxic megacolon?

➢ Total or subsegmental nonobstructive colonic dilation with systemic toxicity
  ▪ Life threatening condition

482. What radiology findings can be seen with toxic megacolon?

➢ Colonic dilation
  ▪ >6 cm

## Colorectal Cancer

483. At what age does colorectal cancer generally occur?

➢ Age >50 years

484. What are suspicious signs and symptoms of colorectal cancer?
> Unintentional weight loss
> GI bleed
> Anemia
> Change in bowel habits

485. What do most colorectal cancers arise from?
> Adenomatous polyps

## Constipation

486. What is an assessment tool used to help characterize stool consistencies?
> The Bristol stool chart

487. What are some treatment options for constipation?
> Lifestyle modifications – increased water and fiber
> Osmotic laxatives (polyethylene glycol, lactulose)
> Bulk-forming laxatives (psyllium, methylcellulose
> Stimulant laxatives (magnesium citrate, Bisacodyl)

## Hemorrhoids

488. What are the most common symptoms of internal, external, and thrombosed hemorrhoids?
> Internal: Painless, bright red rectal bleeding that occurs after defecation
> External: Anal irritation, pruritus, palpable nodule, often asymptomatic

➤ Thrombosed: Painful, edematous external hemorrhoid

489. What methods are considered conservative management for hemorrhoids?

➤ Increase fluids
➤ High-fiber diet (20-30 g/day)
➤ Bulk-forming laxatives
➤ Topical analgesia
➤ Sitz baths
➤ Topical analgesics or hydrocortisone

490. What are some options for management of hemorrhoids that are chronically protruding, irreducible, or have failed conservative therapy?

➤ Sclerotherapy
➤ Rubber-band ligation
➤ Hemorrhoidectomy

## Anal Fissure

491. What is an anal fissure?

➤ Painful, linear cracks in the lining of the anal canal

492. What is the hallmark symptom of anal fissure?

➤ Severe degree of anal pain
  ▪ Increases with defecation

## Anorectal Fistula

493. What diseases/conditions are anorectal fistulas commonly associated with?

➤ Crohn's disease

➤ Constipation

## *Irritable Bowel Syndrome (IBS)*

494. What is IBS?
   ➤ "Functional" gastrointestinal disorder associated with chronic abdominal pain and altered bowel habits

495. What are the common symptoms of irritable bowel syndrome (IBS)? What criteria is used to categorize them?
   ➤ Changes in stool frequency and form (constipation, diarrhea, or mixed), abdominal pain related to defecation, flatulence, bloating, tenesmus, mucous in stool, fecal/urinary incontinence
   ➤ Rome IV criteria

496. What is the treatment for IBS?
   ➤ Lifestyle modifications: increased exercise
   ➤ Low FODMAP diet
   ➤ Probiotics/Prebiotics
   ➤ Symptomatic treatment of diarrhea or constipation
   ➤ TCAs/SSRIs/SNRIs

## *Mesenteric Ischemia*

497. What is the most common cause of acute mesenteric ischemia? What is the classic presentation?
   ➤ Arterial emboli secondary to atrial fibrillation

> Sudden onset abdominal pain out of proportion to exam, blood in stool, hyper-defecation

498. What is the test of choice to confirm acute mesenteric ischemia?

> CTA aorta
> CTA abdomen/pelvis

499. What is the most common vessel involved in acute mesenteric ischemia?

> Superior mesenteric artery (SMA)

500. What are the treatment options for acute mesenteric ischemia?

> NPO
> NG decompression
> IV fluids
> IV antibiotics
> Analgesia
> Surgical revascularization/assess for bowel viability

## Large Bowel Obstruction

501. What is the most common cause of large bowel obstruction?

> Colorectal cancer

502. What are the different types of colonic polyps? Which is most common? Most worrisome?

> Villous – most worrisome, least common
> Tubulovillous
> Tubular – most common
> Hyperplastic – least worrisome

## *Esophageal Disorders*

### *GERD*

503. What is gastroesophageal reflux disease (GERD)?
    ➤ The reflux of stomach acid into the esophagus
      due to lower esophageal sphincter (LES)
      insufficiency

504. What are the treatment options for GERD?
    ➤ Lifestyle modifications – avoid spicy/citrus
      foods, alcohol, caffeine and chocolate, avoid
      laying down within 2 hours of eating, weight loss,
      avoid tobacco/nicotine, elevate head of bed
    ➤ Antacids
    ➤ H2 blockers
    ➤ PPIs
    ➤ Surgery – fundoplication

505. What types of studies are performed in patients
with GERD symptoms refractory to PPIs?
    ➤ pH testing
    ➤ Esophageal motility testing – barium
      swallow/manometry
    ➤ Endoscopy with biopsy

### *Esophagitis*

506. What are the characteristic findings of candida,
HSV, CMV, and HIV esophagitis seen on endoscopy?
    ➤ Candida – white mucosal plaque-like lesions
    ➤ HSV – well circumscribed volcanic-like ulcers
    ➤ CMV/HIV – large shallow ulcers or erosions

507. What is a rare esophageal motor disorder that causes dysphagia to solids and liquids?

> Achalasia

508. What is the classic finding on barium swallow in achalasia?

> "Bird's beak" esophagus

## *Barrett Esophagus*

509. What is Barret esophagus?

> Metaplastic change to the cells in the lower portion of the esophagus to resemble intestinal mucosa

510. Barrett esophagus is most commonly a complication of what condition? Patients are at risk for developing what type of cancer?

> Severe reflux esophagitis
> Esophageal adenocarcinoma

511. How is Barrett's Esophagus diagnosed?

> Upper endoscopy with biopsy

## *Mallory-Weiss Tears*

512. What is a Mallory-Weiss tear? How does it typically present?

> Longitudinal mucosal lacerations in the distal esophagus/proximal stomach caused by forceful retching
> Hematemesis immediately after repeated forceful retching/vomiting often associated with alcohol use

513. What is a Zenker diverticulum? What are the signs and symptoms?

> Acquired, pulsion-type, false diverticulum of mucosal and submucosal layers of the proximal posterior esophagus

> Halitosis, regurgitation of undigested food or pills, dysphagia, gurgling sounds with swallowing

## *Esophageal Varices*

514. What are esophageal varices?

> Enlarged veins in the esophagus from obstructed outflow (portal vein)

515. Who is at risk for developing esophageal varices? What is the treatment for bleeding esophageal varices?

> Risk factors: Cirrhosis of the liver, portal hypertension, advanced liver disease (Child Pugh Class B or C)

> Transfusion, octreotide, PPI, ceftriaxone, endoscopy (band ligation or sclerotherapy), transjugular intrahepatic portosystemic shunt (TIPS)

516. What are the most common risk factors for variceal hemorrhage?

> Variceal size (larger more likely), red wale sign seen on endoscopy, and decompensated cirrhosis

517. In a patient with varices who have never bled what are the two approaches to primary prophylaxis?

> Variceal banding or non-selective beta-blockers

# *Gastric Disorders*

## *Gastritis*

518. What is gastritis?
> ➤ Inflammation of the gastric mucosa

519. What are some common causes of peptic ulcers?
> ➤ H. pylori
> ➤ NSAIDs
> ➤ Alcohol
> ➤ Smoking
> ➤ Caffeine
> ➤ Stress
> ➤ Gastrinoma

## *Peptic Ulcer Disease*

520. What is the most common type of peptic ulcer disease?
> ➤ Duodenal Ulcers

521. How can you differentiate a gastric ulcer from a duodenal ulcer based on symptoms?
> ➤ Gastric – worse shorty after eating, increased pain with eating
> ➤ Duodenal – worse several hours after eating, pain improved with eating

522. What are the ways to test for H. pylori infections?
> ➤ Stool antigen testing, urease breath testing, and biopsy

523. What pharmacological therapeutic combinations are first line therapy for H. pylori with low risk of resistance?

> Triple therapy: Proton pump inhibitor and two antibiotics

## *Pyloric Stenosis*

524. What are the most common symptoms of pyloric stenosis in an infant?
> Projectile, non-bilious, vomiting after feeding
> Palpable "olive-like" mass in the right lower quadrant of the abdomen

525. What is the best test to diagnose pyloric stenosis?
> Ultrasound

# *Hepatic Disorders*

## *Hepatitis*

526. What is the method of transmission of each type of hepatitis?
> Hepatitis A – fecal/oral
> Hepatitis B – parenteral
> Hepatitis C – parenteral
> Hepatitis D – parenteral
> Hepatitis E – fecal/oral

527. Which types of hepatitis have a chronic form?
> Hepatitis B, C, and D

528. What are some signs and symptoms of viral hepatitis?
> Fever, chills, nausea, vomiting, RUQ pain, jaundice, dark tea-colored urine, clay-colored stools, diarrhea (hepatitis A)

529. Which hepatotropic virus commonly found in the U.S. is the only virus not preventable through vaccination?

> Hepatitis C

530. What are the common modes of transmission of hepatitis B and C?

> IV drug use, tattoos and body piercings, vertical transmission, blood transfusions, sex

531. An AST/ALT ratio greater than 2 is suspicious for which type of hepatitis?

> Alcoholic hepatitis

## Nonalcoholic Fatty Liver Disease (NAFLD)

532. What are common conditions that are high risk factors for the development of nonalcoholic fatty liver disease (NAFLD)?

> Obesity, type 2 diabetes, dyslipidemia, polycystic ovarian syndrome

## Ascites

533. What is the Model for End-stage Liver Disease (MELD)?

> Prognostic scoring model for prediction mortality related to cirrhosis over the subsequent 3 months

534. What is the differential diagnosis for ascites other than cirrhosis?

> Nephrotic syndrome, tuberculosis, heart failure, malignancy

535. What is the recommended diet for patients with cirrhosis?

> Dietary sodium restrictions of <2000 mg/day

536. What are the most common causes of acute hepatic encephalopathy in patients with cirrhosis?

> Infections, GI bleeding, constipation, opioid use, over diuresis

537. What may be the only sign of peritoneal infection in patients with cirrhosis?

> Fever

538. When paracentesis is performed on patients with ascites, what is diagnostic of bacterial peritonitis?

> Elevated WBC (≥ 250 cells/mm3) with >50% being absolute polymorphonuclear neutrophils (PMN),
> Positive ascitic fluid bacterial cultures

539. In patients with cirrhosis, upper endoscopy is recommended to screen for what?

> Varices

## *Acute Liver Failure*

540. What is the definition of acute liver failure (ALF)?

> Coagulation abnormalities (INR ≥1.5) and any degree of mental alteration in patients without cirrhosis and illness duration <26 weeks

541. What is the leading cause of ALF in the United States?

> Acetaminophen toxicity

## _Portal Hypertension_

542. What is portal hypertension? What is the most common cause? What are some common manifestations?

> ➤ Pressure in the portal vein exceeds the pressure of the IVC, resistance to portal blood flow
> ➤ Most common – cirrhosis of the liver
> ➤ Manifestations – ascites, esophageal varices, hepatic encephalopathy, splenomegaly, abdominal wall collateral vessels, thrombocytopenia, spider angiomas, gynecomastia

543. What is the surgical procedure used to treat portal hypertension?

> ➤ Transjugular intrahepatic portosystemic shunt (TIPS)

# _Pancreatic Disorders_

## _Acute Pancreatitis_

544. What are the most common causes of acute pancreatitis?

> ➤ Gallstones
> ➤ Alcohol
> ➤ Hypertriglyceridemia

545. What are classic symptoms for acute pancreatitis?

> ➤ Severe epigastrium and/or periumbilical abdominal pain that radiates to back with associated nausea and vomiting

546. What are two late findings on physical exam that can indicate the presence of hemorrhagic pancreatitis?

➤ Cullen's sign: Periumbilical ecchymosis

➤ Grey-Turner's sign: Flank ecchymosis

547. What blood tests are used to diagnose acute pancreatitis?

➤ Elevated lipase (3x the upper limit of normal)

➤ Elevated amylase

548. What scoring system is used to predict the mortality of a patient with acute pancreatitis?

➤ Ranson's Criteria

▪ Age >55

▪ LDH >350 U/L

▪ AST >250 U/L

▪ WBC >16,000/mm$^3$

▪ Glucose >200mg/dL

549. What are the main treatment options for gallstone pancreatitis?

➤ ERCP

➤ Cholecystectomy

550. What complications are associated with acute pancreatitis?

➤ Pancreatic necrosis (with or without infection)

➤ Pseudocyst

➤ Pancreatic abscess

➤ Organ failure (SIRS, respiratory failure, shock, renal failure)

551. What serum triglyceride level is required for the diagnosis of hypertriglyceridemia induced pancreatitis?

➤ >1000 mg/dL

## *Hernias*

552. What is a hernia?
> Protrusion, bulge, or projection of part of an organ through the wall of muscle or tissue that normally contains it

553. What is the difference between a reducible, incarcerated, and strangulated hernia?
> Reducible: Ability to return the hernia sac and contents to anatomic position
> Incarcerated: Hernia that cannot be reduced, painful
> Strangulated: An incarcerated hernia that has become ischemic due to restricted blood flow

554. Which type of hernias are at greatest risk of complication?
> Femoral hernias

555. What is the most common type of abdominal hernia? What is the most common cause?
> Indirect inguinal hernia
> Patent processus vaginalis (congenital)

## *Infectious Diarrhea*

### *Gastroenteritis*

556. What are the classic symptoms of gastroenteritis?
> Abdominal pain, nausea, vomiting, diarrhea, +/- fever

557. What are some common causes of gastroenteritis?
> Viral (most common) – Norovirus, Rotavirus, Adenoviruses, Astrovirus

➢ Bacterial – S. aureus, Salmonella, Shigella, Enterohemorrhagic E. coli, Campylobacter, Yersinia

➢ Parasitic – Entamoeba histolytica, Giardia, Cryptosporidium

## *Clostridium Difficile (C. Diff)*

558. What is the initial treatment for C. Diff?
➢ Cessation of inciting antibiotic as soon as possible
➢ Infection control (ie. contact precautions & hand hygiene)

559. What antibiotics are used to treat C. Diff infection?
➢ Vancomycin
➢ Fidaxomicin
➢ Metronidazole

## Miscellaneous

560. What is a congenital motor disorder of the gut that is typically diagnosed in neonates who present with distal intestinal obstruction, abdominal distention, bilious emesis, and failure to pass stool?
➢ Hirschsprung disease (HD)

561. Which patients are at risk increased risk for Hirschsprung disease?
➢ Trisomy 21 (Down syndrome)

562. What disorder is caused by a deficiency of phenylalanine hydroxylase which can lead to severe

irreversible mental retardation if untreated? When does screening for the exam occur?

> ➤ Phenylketonuria (PKU)
> ➤ Federally mandated test completed at least 48 hours after birth

563. What defines infant colic?

> ➤ Crying for ≥**3** hours per day for no apparent reason,
> ➤ ≥**3** days per week, and
> ➤ <**3** months old
>> ▪ Remember: **"Rule of 3's"**

# 5

---

# ENDOCRINE SYSTEM

## *Diabetes Mellitus*

564. What are the classic signs and symptoms associated with diabetes mellitus?

> Polydipsia, polyuria, polyphagia

565. What are the differences in time of onset between diabetes mellitus type I and type II?

> Type I – early onset (typically in childhood/adolescence)
> Type II – late onset (typically later in life)

566. What are the differences in pathophysiology between diabetes mellitus type I and type II?

> Type I – insulinopenia
> Type II – overproduction of insulin and insulin resistance

567. What are the risk factors for diabetes mellitus type I and type II?

> Type I – family history, race (Caucasian)
> Type II – overweight/obese, family history, sedentary lifestyle, history of gestational diabetes, race (African American, Pacific Islander, Latin American, Alaska Native, Asian American)

568. What are some signs and symptoms of insulin resistance?

> Acanthosis nigricans, hypertension, dyslipidemia, PCOS, obesity

569. What glucose values for each of the three primary screening tests meet criteria for the diagnosis of diabetes?

> Two-hour oral glucose tolerance test: ≥200 mg/dL

> Hemoglobin A1c: ≥6.5%
> Impaired fasting glucose: ≥126 mg/dL

570. What does hemoglobin A1c measure?

> Blood glucose control over the past 3 months

571. What is the first line medication used in the treatment of type I diabetes mellitus?

> Insulin – basal and bolus

572. What important side effect is associated with insulin administration?

> Hypoglycemia

573. What is the first line approach in the treatment of type 2 diabetes mellitus per the American Diabetes Association?

> Lifestyle modification (ie. diet, weight reduction, exercise) and metformin

574. What are the first line pharmacologic therapies for patients with type 2 diabetes mellitus and cardiovascular disease per the American Diabetes Association?

> GLP-1 receptor agonists (ie. liraglutide, dulaglutide, semaglutide, exenatide)
> SGLT2 inhibitors (ie. empagliflozin, dapagliflozin, canagliflozin)

575. What are some ways to improve gastrointestinal intolerance of metformin?

> Slow titration, take medication with food, changing to extended-release form

576. What is a potential adverse event of metformin that commonly prompts discontinuation of the medication during an in-patient hospitalization?

> Lactic acidosis

577. When is metformin therapy contraindicated?

> eGFR <30 mL/min/1.73 m²

578. What are some complications of diabetes mellitus?

> Cardiovascular disease/coronary artery disease
> Cerebrovascular disease
> Peripheral vascular disease
> Nephropathy – microalbuminuria
> Neuropathy – stocking-glove pattern
> Retinopathy – cotton-wool spots

579. What is Kussmaul's breathing?

> Deep, rapid breathing pattern that is associated with metabolic acidosis

580. What medical emergency causes hyperglycemia, ketonuria, and acidosis?

> Diabetic ketoacidosis

581. What is the difference between Diabetic Ketoacidosis (DKA) and Hyperosmolar Hyperglycemic State (HHS)?

> DKA – more common in type 1 diabetics, profound metabolic acidosis
> HHS – more common in type 2 diabetics, profoundly elevated blood glucose

582. What are findings seen in hyperosmolar hyperglycemic state (HHS)?

> More common with type II diabetics
> Marked hyperglycemia (plasma glucose >600)
> Hyperosmolality (serum osmolality >330)
> Severe dehydration

> Commonly without ketosis (or with slight ketosis)

583. What are common precipitants of diabetic ketoacidosis (DKA)?

> Infections, infarctions, alcohol and drug intoxication, nonadherence to insulin, pancreatitis

584. What electrolyte is most commonly depleted in DKA or HHS due to urinary loss and GI upset?

> Potassium

585. What is the treatment for DKA?

> Regular Insulin IV drip
  - Usually requires ICU admission
> Potassium replacement (if necessary)
> IV fluids
> Bicarbonate
  - Controversial, given if arterial pH <6.9

586. What is the treatment for HHS?

> Admission, Insulin, IV fluids

## *Thyroid Disorders*

### *Hypothyroidism*

587. What is the most sensitive test to detect primary hypo or hyperthyroidism?

> TSH

588. What are the classic signs and symptoms associated with hypothyroidism?

> Cold intolerance, weight gain, dry skin, fatigue, constipation, hyporeflexia

589. What are the most common etiologies of hypothyroidism?

> Primary (most common)
> Hashimoto's thyroiditis
> Radioactive iodine
> Radiation therapy

590. What is the typical pattern of TSH and free T4 in subclinical hypothyroidism? Hypothyroidism?

> Subclinical hypothyroidism:
  - Elevated TSH
  - Normal free T4
> Hypothyroidism:
  - Elevated TSH
  - Decreased free T4

591. What is the first-line pharmacologic treatment for hypothyroidism?

> Levothyroxine

592. What antiarrhythmic medication is a common cause of secondary hypothyroidism?

> Amiodarone


## _Hyperthyroidism_

593. What are the common causes of hyperthyroidism?

> Grave's disease
> Single or multinodular goiter
> Thyroiditis
> TSH secreting pituitary tumor

594. What are the classic signs and symptoms associated with hyperthyroidism?

> Heat intolerance, weight loss, tachycardia, palpitations, anxiety, pretibial myxedema, hyperreflexia

595. What is the most common cause for primary hyperthyroidism?
> Grave's Disease

596. What is the most common physical exam findings in Graves ophthalmopathy?
> Exophthalmos

597. What are some common cardiovascular manifestations seen with hyperthyroidism?
> Sinus Tachycardia
> Palpitations
> SVT (occasionally)
> A. fib
  - Usually patients >50 years old

598. If a goiter is palpated on physical exam, what studies should be obtained?
> TSH
> Thyroid ultrasound

599. What is the drug of choice to treat symptomatic palpitations or tachycardia in patients with hyperthyroidism?
> Propranolol

600. What are the treatment options for hyperthyroidism? What is the drug of choice in pregnancy?
> Methimazole
> **P**TU (**P**regnancy)
> Radioactive iodine ablation
> Thyroidectomy

601. What are common side effects of antithyroid drugs?

➢ Rash
➢ Urticaria
➢ Fever
➢ Arthralgia

602. What are signs and symptoms of thyroid storm?
➢ Hyperpyrexia (104-106 is common)
➢ Altered mental status (ie. restlessness, agitation, confusion)
➢ Cardiovascular dysfunction (ie. severe tachycardia, CHF, a. fib)
➢ Nausea, vomiting, diarrhea
➢ Elevation of free T4 and/or T3
➢ Suppression of TSH

603. What is the most common cause of myxedema crisis?
➢ Profound hypothyroidism

604. What are the common signs and symptoms of myxedema coma?
➢ AMS, hypothermia, bradycardia, hypotension, peripheral edema, urinary retention

605. How is myxedema coma treated?
➢ Supportive care
➢ IV T3/T4
➢ IV corticosteroids

## *Thyroiditis*

606. What condition is caused by autoimmune destruction of thyrocytes and is the most common cause of hypothyroidism?
➢ Hashimoto thyroiditis

607. What is the most common cause of painful thyroiditis?

  > DeQuervain's (viral infection)

608. What thyroid antibody is commonly elevated in Hashimoto's thyroiditis?

  > Antithyroid peroxidase (TPO)

609. What are the common causes of painless thyroiditis?

  > Autoimmune
  > Lymphocytic
  > Postpartum
  > Radiation

## Adrenal Disorders

### Adrenal Insufficiency

610. What is the location of disease in primary adrenal insufficiency (AI)? In secondary AI?

  > Primary: Adrenocortical disease (Addison's disease)
  > Secondary: Pituitary gland

611. What are the most common clinical manifestations of primary and secondary AI?

  > Weakness, fatigue, orthostatic hypotension, anorexia, weight loss

612. What is the classic dermatologic manifestation of primary AI?

  > Hyperpigmentation seen in mucous membranes, nipples, and creases

613. What levels of morning serum cortisol can effectively rule in AI? Rule out AI?

> Rules it in: <3 ug/dL
> Rules it out: >18 ug/dL

614. What is the most common diagnostic test to evaluate for AI?

> ACTH (cosyntropin) stimulation test

615. What are laboratory findings for Addison's Disease?

> Hypoglycemia
> Hyponatremia
> Hyperkalemia

616. What test is used to differentiate between primary and secondary adrenal insufficiency?

> Morning ACTH
  - Primary adrenal insufficiency – high
  - Secondary adrenal insufficiency – low/normal

617. What is the treatment for primary and secondary adrenal insufficiency?

> Primary: Glucocorticoids (ie. hydrocortisone) and mineralocorticoids (ie. fludrocortisone)
> Secondary: Glucocorticoids only (ie. hydrocortisone)

618. What are the typical signs and symptoms associated with adrenal crisis?

> Fever, abdominal/chest pain, hypotension (refractory to IV fluids/vasopressors)

619. What is the difference between Cushing's syndrome and Cushing's disease? What is the most common cause of each?

> Syndrome: Cortisol excess
  - Exogenous glucocorticoids

> Disease: Pituitary ACTH hypersecretion causing
  Cushing's syndrome
  - Pituitary adenoma

620. What are laboratory findings for Cushing Syndrome?

> Hyperglycemia
> Hypernatremia
> Hypokalemia

621. What are the classic signs and symptoms associated with Cushing syndrome?

> Obesity, buffalo hump, moon facies, pigmented striae, hypertension

622. What tests are used to diagnose hypercortisolism?

> Dexamethasone suppression tests
  - Low dose – no suppression of cortisol
  - High dose – suppression of cortisol if pituitary/adrenal lesion, but not ectopic (SCLC)

623. What is the treatment for Cushing syndrome secondary to exogenous steroid use?

> Steroid taper


## _Pheochromocytoma_

624. What is a pheochromocytoma?

> Tumor of the adrenal medulla causing increased catecholamine secretions

625. What is the classic presentation of a pheochromocytoma?

> **P**alpitations
> **H**eadache

> E̲xcessive sweating
  - Remember: "**PHE**"
> Other symptoms: fever, hypertension, tachycardia, AMS

626. What labs are used to diagnose pheochromocytoma?

> Free metanephrines and catecholamines
> 24-hour urine metanephrines and catecholamines

## *Parathyroid Disorders*

627. What hormone is the key regulator of calcium and phosphate homeostasis?

> Parathyroid hormone (PTH)

628. What is the main calcium binding protein?

> Albumin

629. What is the most common cause of hypercalcemia?

> Hyperparathyroidism secondary to an adenoma

630. What malignancies classically cause an increase in hypercalcemia?

> Breast
> Lung
> Multiple myeloma
> Renal cell

631. What are some signs and symptoms associated with hypercalcemia?

> "Stones, bones, groans, psychiatric moans"
  - Stones – kidney stones
  - Bones – osteopenia, osteoporosis, MSK pain

- Groans – abdominal pain, nausea, vomiting, constipation
- Psychiatric moans – decreased cognitive function, lethargy

632. What is the most common cause of hypoparathyroidism?

> Thyroid surgery (thyroidectomy)

633. How does hypoparathyroidism present?

> Symptoms of hypocalcemia – perioral tingling, paresthesias, tetany
  - Chvostek's sign – facial twitching when tapping on facial nerve
  - Trousseau's sign – carpal spasm following the inflation of a blood pressure cuff

## *Pituitary Disorders*

634. What is the most common cause of acromegaly?

> Pituitary adenoma

635. Deficiency of growth hormone (GH) leads to what disorder?

> Pituitary dwarfism

636. What is the most common type of pituitary adenoma?

> Prolactinoma

637. What is the best imaging modality to identify a pituitary adenoma?

> MRI

## *Diabetes Insipidus*

638. What are some common causes of diabetes insipidus (DI)?
> ➤ CNS disorders/trauma
> ➤ Medications
> ➤ Renal disease

639. What are the two types of DI?
> ➤ Central
> ➤ Nephrogenic

640. What are the classic signs and symptoms of DI?
> ➤ Polyuria and polydipsia

641. What lab abnormalities are seen in DI?
> ➤ Increased serum osmolality
> ➤ Decreased urine osmolality

642. What test is used to differentiate between central and nephrogenic DI?
> ➤ Water deprivation test + desmopressin
>  ▪ Central – increase in urine osmolality
>  ▪ Nephrogenic – no change in urine osmolality

643. What are the treatment options for central DI?
> ➤ Desmopressin (DDAVP)
> ➤ Indomethacin

644. What are the treatment options for nephrogenic DI?
> ➤ Hydrochlorothiazide
> ➤ Indomethacin

# 6

## DERMATOLOGIC SYSTEM

## *Acneiform Eruptions*

645. How does acne vulgaris present?
- Open comedones – noninflammatory blackheads
- Closed comedones – noninflammatory whiteheads
- Papules – inflammatory with no pus
- Pustules – inflammatory with pus
- Cysts/nodules

646. What are the treatment options for acne vulgaris?
- Topical
  - Salicylic acid
  - Benzoyl peroxide
  - Retinoids
  - Antibiotics
- Oral (PO)
  - Antibiotics (ie. tetracyclines)
  - Spironolactone
  - Isotretinoin
  - Contraceptives

647. What are triggers of folliculitis?
- Tight clothing/friction
- Hot tubs
- Shaving

648. What is rosacea? What are the clinical features? What is the treatment?
- Chronic, relapsing inflammatory skin disorder of the central face
- Facial erythema, telangiectasias, inflammatory papules/pustules

> Treatment – topical metronidazole, PO
antibiotics (tetracyclines), sulfur

## Desquamation

649. What are common causes of erythema multiforme
(EM)? How does it present? How is it treated?

> Viral (HSV), medications (NSAIDs, sulfa drugs,
anti-epileptics)
> Symmetric target lesions on acral sites that
progress centripetally
> Treatment – supportive care
  - PO antihistamines
  - Topical corticosteroids

650. What are some common causes of Steven-
Johnson Syndrome (SJS)?

> Medications – antibiotics (penicillin, sulfa-
containing drugs), NSAIDs, anti-epileptics,
allopurinol
> Infection
> Malignancy
> Idiopathic

651. What is the difference between SJS and Toxic
Epidermal Necrolysis (TEN)? Where should they both
be admitted to?

> SJS – <10% BSA
> TEN – >30% BSA
> Burn center

## Hair & Nails

652. What is alopecia areata caused by? How does it present?
  ➢ Autoimmune dysfunction
  ➢ Round, patchy hair loss with "exclamation point" hairs

653. What is onychomycosis?
  ➢ Fungal infection of the nail

654. What is the difference between paronychia and felon? What is the most common organism associated with both of them?
  ➢ Paronychia – infection of the nail fold
  ➢ Felon – infection of the fingertip pulp
  ➢ S. aureus

655. What is the treatment for a painful subungual hematoma with intact nail folds?
  ➢ Trephination

## Exanthems

656. What characteristic rash is associated with erythema infectiosum?
  ➢ "Slapped cheek" – flushed cheeks, macular → lacy rash

657. What is the characteristic rash associated with hand, foot, and mouth disease? What are the most common pathogens? What is the medical management?
  ➢ Vesicular lesions on the mouth, hands, and feet (may include palms and soles)
  ➢ Coxsackievirus and Enterovirus

> Supportive care - ibuprofen or acetaminophen, hydration

658. What are Koplik spots? What disease are they associated with?

> Small lesions on the buccal mucosa with red base and white/grey specks
> Measles

## Infectious Diseases

659. What is cellulitis? What are the most common organisms involved? What is the treatment?

> Inflammation/infection of the epidermis and subcutaneous tissue
> Staphylococcus and Streptococcus species
> Treatment - PO antibiotics
  - Consider IV if no resolution on PO antibiotics

660. What differentiates cellulitis from an abscess?

> Cellulitis – erythema with no fluctuance or drainage
> Abscess – fluctuance with possible drainage

661. What is a chronic skin infection that develops a cyst or abscess at or near the upper part of the natal cleft between the buttocks?

> Pilonidal disease

662. How does impetigo present? What is the treatment?

> Honey crusted vesicles +/- bullae
> Treatment – topical mupirocin or PO antibiotics (cephalexin)

663. What is necrotizing fasciitis?

> Life threatening infection that spreads along soft tissue planes

664. What is the classic presentation associated with candidal dermatitis? What is the treatment?

> "Beefy-red" rash with satellite lesions
> Treatment – topical/PO antifungals

665. What are the types of tinea infections?

> Tinea capitis – hair shafts/scalp
> Tinea corporis – body
> Tinea cruris – skin folds (jock itch)
> Tinea pedis – feet (athlete's foot)

666. What fungal skin infection presents with multiple hypo/hyperpigmented discrete macules, scaly lesions to the chest, back, and arms?

> Tinea versicolor

667. How does seborrheic dermatitis present?

> Infants – "cradle cap"
> Adults – greasy, yellow scales/dandruff
  - Often presents in eyebrows, beards and the nasal groove

668. How does lice infestation present? What medications may be used to treat it?

> Pruritus, visualization of lice/nits
> Treatment – permethrin, ivermectin

669. How does scabies infestation present? What medications may be used to treat it?

> Pruritic rash, burrows in the web spaces
> Treatment – permethrin, ivermectin

670. How is the rash associated with varicella zoster virus (VZV) described?

> Grouped vesicles on an erythematous base ("dew drops on a rose petal") that erupt in crops then crust over

671. How is the rash associated with shingles (herpes zoster) described? How is it treated? What is the long-term risk of delayed antiviral treatment?

> Grouped vesicles on an erythematous base that do not cross midline and stay in unilateral dermatomal distribution
> Treatment – antiviral therapy and analgesia
> Postherpetic neuralgia

672. How does a meningococcal rash usually present?

> Petechial rash
> Discrete lesions 1-2mm in diameter
> Usually located to trunk and lower extremities

## Neoplasms

673. What is the most common type of skin cancer?

> Basal cell carcinoma

674. What is the number one risk factor for development of skin cancer?

> Chronic UV radiation/sun exposure

675. What is the classic presentation of basal cell carcinoma? What are some treatment options?

> Pink/pearly lesion with rolled edges, central ulceration/depression, superficial telangiectasia
> Treatment – imiquimod, 5-FU, surgical excision, oral vismodegib

676. What is the classic presentation of squamous cell carcinoma (SCC)? What are some treatment options?

> Scaly, erythematous plaque/ulceration
> Treatment – cryotherapy, surgical excision

677. What features increase suspicion that a lesion may be melanoma?

> **A**symmetry
> **B**order irregularity
> **C**olor variation
> **D**iameter (>6 mm)
> **E**volving
>   - Remember: "**ABCDE**"

## *Papulosquamous Disorders*

678. What are some common causes of contact dermatitis? How can it be differentiated from other pruritic rashes?

> Plants (poison ivy/oak), metals (nickel), irritants (soap, water, etc.)
> Localized to areas of exposed skin

679. What is another name for atopic dermatitis? What other conditions is it associated with?

> Eczema
> Atopy triad – eczema, allergic rhinitis, asthma

680. How does atopic dermatitis present?

> Pruritic, erythematous rash on flexural surfaces

681. How does dyshidrosis present?

> Highly pruritic, "tapioca-like" vesicles on fingers/toes

682. How does the rash in pityriasis rosea present? How is it treated?

> "Christmas tree" pattern on the back with salmon-colored herald patch
> Treatment – supportive care

683. How does psoriasis present? How is it treated?

> Erythematous well-demarcated plaques with silvery-scale on extensor surfaces and scalp
> Treatment – topical corticosteroids, vitamin D analogs, UVB therapy, biologics

## Skin Integrity

684. What are the types of thermal burns according to depth?

> First-degree (epidermis) – erythematous, no blisters, painful
> Second-degree (partial thickness dermis)
>   - Superficial (papillary dermis) – thin-walled blisters, painful
>   - Deep (papillary and reticular dermis) – thick-walled blisters, painful
> Third-degree (full-thickness dermis) – white, charred, painless
> Fourth-degree (subQ tissue, muscle, fascia, bone) – eschar, painless

685. What is the rule of 9s?

> Rule for estimating the surface are involvement of a burn
>   - Head – 9% (anterior 4.5%, posterior 4.5%)
>   - Chest – 9%
>   - Stomach – 9%
>   - Upper back – 9%

- Lower back – 9%
- Each arm – 9% (anterior 4.5%, posterior 4.5%)
- Each leg – 18% (anterior 9%, posterior 9%)
- Genitalia – 1%

686. What formula is used to calculate fluid resuscitation needs in a thermal burn patient? What is the preferred fluid?

> Parkland formula – ½ in the first 8 hours, remaining ½ over the next 16 hours
> - 4 mL x kg x % total body surface area
> Lactated Ringers

687. What are the two broad categories of sutures?

> Absorbable – vicryl, monocryl, PDS, chromic gut
> Nonabsorbable – prolene, nylon, silk

688. What is the staging system used to describe pressure ulcers?

> Stage I – non-blanching erythema that blanches, no loss of skin
> Stage II – partial thickness loss of skin
> Stage III – full thickness loss of skin
> Stage IV – full thickness loss of skin with exposure of subQ tissue, muscle, fascia, bone

689. What is the preferred antibiotic for prophylaxis following an animal bite?

> Amoxicillin-clavulanate

## Other Dermatologic Disorders

690. What disorders is acanthosis nigricans associated with? How does it present?

> Insulin resistance (obesity, DM), PCOS, malignancy
> Hyperpigmentation of the skin folds with velvety appearance, skin appears dirty

691. What is the difference between melasma and vitiligo?

> Melasma – hyperpigmentation
> Vitiligo – depigmentation

692. Where does hidradenitis suppurativa typically occur? How does it present? What are the treatment options?

> Axillae, breast folds, groin, perineum, buttocks
> Draining sinus tracts or recurrent abscesses
> Treatment – weight reduction, smoking cessation, hygiene, topical/PO antibiotics, intralesional steroid injections, biologics, excision

693. What is the difference between an epidermal inclusion cyst (EIC) and a lipoma?

> EIC – firm, mobile mass with central punctum, contents surrounded by cyst wall
> Lipoma – soft, mobile mass composed of adipose cells with no cyst wall

694. What are the risk factors for pilonidal disease? What are the treatment options?

> Deep gluteal cleft, hirsutism, friction
> Treatment – wound care, Sitz baths, hygiene, I&D, surgical excision

695. What type of hypersensitivity reaction is urticaria? What are some of the most common causes? How is it treated?

> IgE mediated
> Medications, food, and insect bites
> H1 blocker
  - 1$^{st}$ generation – diphenhydramine
  - 2$^{nd}$ generation – cetirizine, loratadine

696. Severe urticaria with mucosal involvement and difficulty swallowing should raise suspicion for what? What is the initial treatment?

> Anaphylaxis
> Treatment – IM epinephrine

697. What are causes of a rash occurring on the palms and soles?

> Kawasaki disease
> Coxsackie
> Rocky Mountain Spotted Fever
> Syphilis
> SJS/TEN
> Erythema Multiforme

698. How does the rash associated with Kawasaki disease present? What are other common symptoms associated with it? What is the treatment?

> Polymorphous exanthem with associated erythema, induration, swelling, and desquamatization of the hands/feet
> Fever >5 days, bilateral conjunctivitis, cervical lymphadenopathy, oral changes (swelling/erythema, strawberry tongue)
> Treatment – IVIG and aspirin

699. What is the hallmark for the rash associated with Rocky Mountain Spotted Fever?

> Erythematous, blanching rash with macules that become petechial and purpuric
  - Usually starts on the extremities/wrist/ankles and then moves to trunk

700. What is erythema migrans?
  > A red skin lesion at the site of a tick bite
    - Expands slowly over the course of days or weeks
    - Often with central clearing (target or bull's eye appearance)
  > Suggestive of early Lyme disease

## Pediatrics

701. What is congenital dermal melanocytosis?
  > Also known as Mongolian spots
  > Benign, congenital, macular blue-gray pigmentation
    - Often located to sacral area and buttock

702. What is milia?
  > White papules seen in neonates, most commonly seen on nose and cheeks
    - Due to retention of keratin and sebaceous material
  > Spontaneously resolves within first 1-2 weeks of life

703. What is Erythema toxicum neonatorum?
  > A common newborn erythematous macular rash with pinpoint, white-yellow papules and pustules

- Occurs within the first few days of life and resolves usually spontaneously within the first week of life

704. What genetic disorder is highly suggestive with the presences of six of more café-au-lait macules? Who should the patient be referred to?

> Neurofibromatosis
> Pediatric neurologist

705. What is a Port Wine Stain? What is the treatment?

> Blanching, pink-red patches present at birth due to congenital capillary malformations
  - Also known as nevus flammeus
> Treatment - pulsed dye laser (PDL) therapy

706. What is a first-line therapy for an uncomplicated infantile hemangioma? Complicated infantile hemangioma?

> Uncomplicated – watchful waiting, majority involute spontaneously after 12 months old
> Complicated – oral propranolol

707. What causes a diffuse erythematous, "sandpaper", blanching rash that is typically accompanied by a strawberry tongue and pharyngitis?

> Scarlet fever

708. What are the clinical features of molluscum contagiosum?

> Firm, dome shaped, flesh-colored papules with central indentation
  - Often 2-5 mm in diameter
  - May occur anywhere on the body except palms and soles

709. What newborn rash presents as a single or multiple blanching, pink-red patches from capillary malformation most commonly located on upper eyelids, upper lip, forehead, or the nap of the neck?

> Nexus simplex (also called macular stain, angel kiss, stork bite)

Dermatologic System

# 7

---

# EYES, EARS,
# NOSE & THROAT

# Eye Disorders

## Conjunctivitis

710. What is the most common cause of conjunctivitis?
> ➤ Adenovirus

711. What are the differences in presentation between viral, bacterial, and allergic conjunctivitis?
> ➤ Viral – watery discharge, preauricular lymphadenopathy, unilateral or bilateral
> ➤ Bacterial – purulent discharge, "glued shut" appearance, may start unilateral then move to contralateral eye
> ➤ Allergic – itching (hallmark symptom), mucoid "stringy" discharge, bilateral + signs/symptoms of allergic rhinitis

712. What are the common causes of infectious conjunctivitis in newborns? At what ages do they occur? What are the signs and symptoms of each?
> ➤ Gonorrhea – 2-7 days old – red eyes, profuse thick pus and swelling of the eyelids
> ➤ Chlamydia – 5-14 days old – mucopurulent or bloody discharge, marked swelling with red, thickened, and friable conjunctivae

713. What prophylactic measure is taken shortly after birth to reduce the risk of gonococcal ophthalmia neonatorum?
> ➤ Erythromycin 0.5% ophthalmic ointment given to all newborns

## *Cataracts*

714. What are cataracts? What are the two types of cataracts?
> ➢ Opacity of the lens
> ➢ Types:
>> ▪ Nuclear (central)
>> ▪ Cortical (on the sides)

715. What are clinical symptoms of cataracts? In what age group is it most common?
> ➢ Painless, halos around lights, difficulty with driving at night (associated with glaring of headlights),
> ➢ Typically occurs in > 60 years old

716. What are risk factors associated with cataracts?
> ➢ Advanced age, smoking, diabetes mellitus, systemic corticosteroid use, UV light exposure, trauma, electric shock, HIV/AIDS

717. What is the treatment for cataracts?
> ➢ Surgical removal of the opacified lens

## *Corneal Ulcer (Keratitis)*

718. What are some risk factors for development of a corneal ulcer (keratitis)? What would you see on exam with fluorescein stain?
> ➢ Contact lens use, trauma, dry eyes
> ➢ Corneal infiltrate, large corneal abrasion

719. What are some serious complications of a corneal ulcer?

> Perforation, stromal necrosis, corneal scarring, vision loss, secondary infection, cataracts, glaucoma
> Consult ophthalmology

## *Herpes Simplex Keratitis*

720. How does herpes simplex keratitis appear on exam with fluorescein stain? What is the treatment?

> Pathognomonic dendritic lesions or geographic ulcers
> Acyclovir 3% ophthalmic ointment is the preferred topical treatment, topical trifluridine

721. What are symptoms associated with herpes simplex keratitis?

> Blurred vision, pain, photophobia, watery ocular discharge, eye redness

722. What is a serious complication of herpes simplex keratitis?

> Blindness

## *Pterygium/Pinguecula*

723. What is the primary difference between pterygium and pinguecula?

> Pterygium – pink triangular tissue growth that spreads onto the cornea, can interfere with vision
>  ▪ Remember: "pTeRY for TRIanglular growth"
> Pinguecula – does not spread onto the cornea, does not interfere with vision

## _Lacrimal Glands_

724. What disease is characterized by inflammation and infection of the lacrimal glands? What is the treatment?

- ➢ Dacryoadenitis - inflammation or infection of the lacrimal gland from which tears are secreted
  - ▪ Dacryocystitis is an infection within the lacrimal drainage system
- ➢ Treatment – warm compresses, antibiotics, consider corticosteroids if inflammatory cause, possible surgical intervention

## _Blepharitis_

725. What is blepharitis? What are the different types of blepharitis?

- ➢ Inflammation, discharge and crusting of the eyelid margins
- ➢ Anterior blepharitis: Inflammation of the base of the eyelashes
- ➢ Posterior blepharitis: Inflammation of the inner portion of the eyelid
  - ▪ Involves abnormal functioning of the meibomian glands
  - ▪ More common type

726. What pathogen is primary associated with anterior blepharitis?

- ➢ Staphylococcus aureus
  - ▪ Women > Men
  - ▪ Associated with contaminated eye makeup

727. What should be suspected for any nonhealing, ulcerative lesion of the eyelids?

> ➤ Basal cell, squamous cell, or meibomian gland carcinoma
> ➤ Autoimmune disease, HIV or other underlying disease process

## *Chalazion/Hordeolum*

728. What is the difference between chalazion and hordeolum? What are their treatments?
> ➤ Chalazion – painless soft tissue swelling due to Meibomian gland obstruction
>   ▪ Treated with warm compresses
> ➤ Hordeolum (stye) – painful infection of the Meibomian glands
>   ▪ Treated with warm compresses and antibiotics (topical or systemic)

## *Nystagmus*

729. How does nystagmus present with peripheral vs. central etiology?
> ➤ Peripheral – unidirectional (can be horizontal or rotatory) nystagmus
> ➤ Central – unidirectional or multidirectional, vertical nystagmus; worsened by fixation of gaze

## *Papilledema*

730. What does papilledema appear on fundoscopic exam? What does it indicate?
> ➤ Swelling of the optic disc with blurred margins
> ➤ Increased intracranial pressure (ICP)

## *Orbital Cellulitis*

731. What is the difference between orbital cellulitis and preseptal cellulitis?
> Orbital cellulitis: Infection involving the tissues posterior to the orbital septum (ie. fat and ocular muscles)
> Preseptal cellulitis (aka periorbital cellulitis): Infection of the soft tissues anterior to the orbital septum

732. What symptoms are usually more suggestive of orbital cellulitis?
> Pain with eye movement, proptosis, restriction of eye movement

733. What are some complications of orbital cellulitis?
> Subperiosteal abscess, orbital abscess, vision loss, cavernous sinus thrombosis, brain abscess, central retinal artery occlusion, meningitis, potentially fatal

## *Macular Degeneration*

734. In the elderly, what is the major cause for gradual, painless, bilateral central vision loss?
> Macular degeneration

735. What is seen on fundoscopic exam with macular degeneration? What test is used to diagnosis it?
> Drusen spots (small yellow or white spots on the retina)
> Amsler grid used to detect early signs of retinal disease

736. What is the difference between wet and dry macular degeneration?

> Wet: Exudative, neovascular, more severe form, can cause vision loss
> Dry: Nonexudative, atrophic, most common, less severe

## *Retinal Detachment*

737. What are common signs and symptoms of retinal detachment?

> Sudden, painless vision loss, flashing lights, floaters, "curtain-like shadow" coming down over visual field
> Requires emergent ophthalmology consult
> Consider verification with handheld ultrasound to look for free-waving or "dancing" retina, appears white on images

## *Retinopathy*

738. What two chronic diseases are associated with the development of retinopathy? How do they appear on fundoscopic exam?

> Diabetes
  ▪ Diabetic retinopathy – wet retina, multiple hemorrhages, extensive edema, microaneurysms, yellow hard exudates, rare flame-shaped hemorrhages, cotton wool spots, abnormal veins
> Hypertension

- Hypertensive retinopathy – dry retina, copper/silver wiring, AV nicking, flame hemorrhages, cotton wool spots, yellow hard exudates

## *Orbital Fracture*

739. What is the most common mechanism of injury for an orbital blowout fracture? What are the common physical exam findings?
  - ➤ Trauma to the face/eye
  - ➤ Swelling, restricted EOMs, diplopia, exophthalmos, hypoesthesia along trigeminal nerve (V2)
    - Check for associated septal hematoma if there is co-existing nasal trauma

## *Corneal Abrasion*

740. What is the best way to visualize a corneal abrasion?
  - ➤ Fluorescein drops in eye with Slit lamp using a cobalt-blue light

741. What type of coverage with antibiotics should be prescribed for corneal abrasions seen in contact wearers?
  - ➤ Pseudomonal coverage
  - ➤ Topical ciprofloxacin or ofloxacin is recommended as first line agents
    - If unable to use fluoroquinolones, consider tobramycin or gentamicin

- Consider topical anesthetic drops in compliant patient for 2-3 days (maximum)

## *Ruptured Globe*

742. What should be done if a ruptured globe is suspected?
  ➢ Emergent ophthalmology consult
  ➢ Avoid any eye manipulation or applying pressure
  ➢ Shield the globe with Fox Shield or Styrofoam cup
  ➢ Elevated HOB
  ➢ May confirm with Seidel Test

## *Hyphema*

743. What is blood seen in the anterior chamber of the eye called?
  ➢ Hyphema
    - Usually caused by blunt trauma
    - Urgent ophthalmology consult

## *Subconjunctival Hemorrhage*

744. What are the causes and treatment for a subconjunctival hemorrhage?
  ➢ Usually occurs spontaneously
  ➢ May be caused by trauma, coughing, sneezing, eye rubbing
  ➢ Treatment: Resolves without any intervention or treatment
  ➢ Does **not** always need CT imaging of head

## *Uveitis*

745. What is uveitis? What are the three types of uveitis?

> Inflammation of the uvea (middle portion of the eye)
> Types:
>> Anterior (involves the iris and ciliary body)
>> Intermediate
>> Posterior (involves the choroid)

746. What are the symptoms and treatment for uveitis?

> Eye pain, blurred vision, photophobia
> Treatment: Topical steroids, cycloplegics
> Ophthalmology consult

## *Central Retinal Artery/Vein Occlusion*

747. What signs and symptoms are associated with central retinal artery occlusion (CRAO)? What would you see on physical exam?

> Sudden, painless, severe vision loss
> Fixed dilated pupil, relevant pupillary defect, "cherry-red spot" on macula seen on fundoscopic exam

748. What are the treatment options for CRAO?

> Digital massage of globe
> $CO_2$ rebreathing techniques
> Reduction of IOP: topical timolol or IV acetazolamide
> Emergent ophthalmology consult

749. What signs and symptoms are associated with central retinal vein occlusion (CRVO)? What would you see on fundoscopic exam?

> Sudden, blurred, painless vision loss
> "Blood and thunder" optic disk edema, diffuse retinal hemorrhages

## Amaurosis Fugax

750. What is amaurosis fugax? What is it commonly associated with?

> Transient visual disturbance described as curtain coming down over visual field
> Transient ischemic attack (TIA)

## Amblyopia

751. What is amblyopia?

> "Lazy eye" – decreased visual acuity in one eye that is not correctable by glasses/contacts

## Glaucoma

752. What is the difference between acute angle closure and open angle glaucoma?

> Acute angle closure glaucoma – acute occlusion of the trabecular meshwork that leads to a sudden elevation of IOP, closed angle between iris and cornea, occurs rapidly, requires immediate medical attention
> Open angle glaucoma – chronic blockage of the trabecular meshwork that leads to chronically

elevated IOP, open angle between iris and cornea, develops slowly and a lifelong condition

753. What are the classic signs and symptoms of acute angle closure glaucoma?

> Severe, unilateral eye pain and loss of vision (commonly associated with entering a dark room or movie theatre)
> Mid-dilated, non-reactive pupil, hazy cornea, halos seen around lights
> Tense globe with finger touch test
> Nausea and vomiting
> Elevated IOP (>21 mmHg)

754. What is the treatment for acute angle closure glaucoma?

> Topical timolol or IV acetazolamide
> IV mannitol
> IV pilocarpine
> Emergent ophthalmology referral

## *Strabismus*

755. What is strabismus?

> Condition of misalignment of the eyes
> May be horizontal, vertical, torsional, or a combination

## *Optic Neuritis*

756. What is optic neuritis? What disease is optic neuritis commonly associated with? What is the classic presentation of optic neuritis?

> Inflammation of the optic nerve

> Multiple sclerosis
> Decreased vision acuity, loss of color vision (red), pain with EOMs

## Foreign Bodies

757. What does a rust ring in the eye indicate?
> Metal foreign body
> Confirm tetanus immunization status
> Examine both eyes, nares and mouth

## Retinoblastoma

758. What is retinoblastoma? What is the classic physical exam finding?
> Rare, malignant intraocular tumor of the retina
  ▪ Most commonly seen in young children
> Unilateral leukocoria (abnormal white pupillary reflex); "cat-eye appearance"

## Miscellaneous

759. What cranial nerves are associated with eye movements?
> Oculomotor (III)
> Trochlear (IV)
> Abducens (VI)

760. What is the difference between miosis and mydriasis?
> Miosis: Constricted pupil
> Mydriasis: Dilated pupil

761. What is Exophthalmos? What disease process is it associated with?

> Protrusion or bulging of the eyeball
  - Also referred to as proptosis
> Grave's Disease

762. What is normal IOP measurements?
> 8 to 21 mmHg
  - >21 mmHg consider open-angle glaucoma

763. What are dendritic lesions? And what are they associated with?
> Linear branching corneal ulcers
> Herpes simplex keratitis

764. What is Seidel Sign? What does it indicate?
> Streaming of fluorescein in a teardrop pattern due to leaking aqueous humor
> Indicates penetrating trauma, ruptured globe

## Ear Disorders

### Cerumen Impaction

765. When should cerumen impactions be removed?
> Symptomatic patients with hearing loss, ear pain, fullness, or itching
> Young children, patients with cognitive impairment, or elderly who are unable to express symptoms

### Otitis Externa

766. What are common physical exam findings seen with otitis externa?
> Pain with palpation of the external ear, tenderness on palpation to tragus, debris and/or

drainage in ear canal, erythema and swelling to ear canal

767. What is the treatment for otitis externa?

> Topical antibiotics (fluoroquinolones)
> Topical steroids (if no perforation)
> Ear wick if edematous

## Malignant Otitis Externa

768. What is malignant otitis externa? What is the most common organism associated with it?

> Invasive external ear infection that spreads from the periauricular tissue to the adjacent bones of the skull and/or TMJ leading to osteomyelitis
> Pseudomonas aeruginosa

769. What are the classic signs and symptoms associated with malignant otitis externa? What is the treatment?

> Fever, pain out of proportion, tenderness at mastoid tip, pain with traction of the pinna, purulent otorrhea, presence of granulation tissue, possible CN involvement (facial nerve dysfunction)
> IV antibiotics, usually requires admission

## Otitis Media

770. What condition commonly precedes acute otitis media (AOM)? What is the most common pathogen associated with it?

> URI
> S. pneumoniae

771. What are the signs and symptoms of AOM? What would you see on physical exam?

> Fever, ear pain, hearing loss
> Erythematous/bulging tympanic membrane (TM) with hypomobility

772. What is the first line antibiotic therapy recommended for acute otitis media?

> Amoxicillin

## Subperichondrial Hematoma

773. What is the common name for subperichondrial hematoma? What is the most common cause? What is the treatment?

> Cauliflower ear
> Blunt trauma
> I&D, pressure dressing, antibiotics

## Foreign Bodies

774. What type of foreign bodies in the ear should not be irrigated?

> Organic foreign bodies (ie. peas)

## Barotrauma

775. What activities is barotrauma associated with? What methods are used to improve symptoms and prevent TM rupture?

> Rapid changes in altitude (ie. flying, diving)
> Auto-insufflation, swallowing, yawning, decongestants

## *Ruptured Tympanic Membrane*

776. What are the typical symptoms for a perforated tympanic member? How does the tympanic member appear on exam?

> ➤ Sudden onset of unilateral ear pain, decreased hearing, otorrhea, then sudden resolution of pain
> ➤ Tear or perforation will be visualized with the otoscopy, bloody otorrhea may also be present

## *Eustachian Tube Dysfunction*

777. What population is more at risk for Eustachian tube (ET) dysfunction? What does this predispose them to?

> ➤ Children – ET is more horizontal
> ➤ Acute otitis media

## *Labyrinthitis*

778. Labyrinthitis is often preceded by what condition? What is the clinical presentation for labyrinthitis?

> ➤ URI
> ➤ Vertigo, nausea, vomiting
>   ▪ Symptoms aggravated by rapid head movement
>   ▪ Tinnitus and hearing loss may also be present

## *Vertigo*

779. What is vertigo? What medications can be used to relieve the symptoms?

> Sensation of movement in the absence of movement
> Vestibular suppressants – antihistamines, benzodiazepines

780. What is the most common form of vertigo?

> Benign paroxysmal positional vertigo (BPPV)

781. What is the cause of benign paroxysmal positional vertigo (BPPV)?

> Otoconia (calcium carbonate crystals present in the utricle) becomes dislodged and moves into the posterior semicircular canal

782. What physical exam maneuver is used to assess for benign paroxysmal positional vertigo (BPPV)? What maneuver is used to treat it?

> Dix-Hallpike maneuver
> Epley maneuver

783. What are common causes of conductive and sensorineural hearing loss?

> Conductive – cerumen impaction, eustachian tube dysfunction, otitis externa
> Sensorineural – presbycusis, acoustic neuroma, acoustic trauma, Meniere's disease

784. What would Rinne and Weber tests show with conductive vs. sensorineural hearing loss?

> Conductive
>   ▪ Rinne – bone > air
>   ▪ Weber – lateralizes to affected ear
> Sensorineural
>   ▪ Rinne – air > bone
>   ▪ Weber – lateralizes to unaffected ear

## *Presbycusis*

785. What is presbycusis? What factors influence the progression of this condition? What is the treatment?
  ➢ Age-related hearing loss
  ➢ Noise trauma (main cause of cochlear damage), genetics, medications, infections
  ➢ Hearing aids

## *Mastoiditis*

786. What condition leads to mastoiditis? What are the signs and symptoms?
  ➢ Untreated/inadequately treated AOM
  ➢ Fever, mastoid erythema/edema, pain with palpation/percussion of the mastoid, protrusion and displacement of the auricle
787. What is the treatment for mastoiditis?
  ➢ IV antibiotics
  ➢ Possible surgical intervention (mastoidectomy)
788. What diagnostic imaging should be ordered if signs and symptoms of mastoiditis are present?
  ➢ CT scan of the temporal bones

## *Meniere's Disease*

789. What are the four common symptoms that may occur simultaneously with Meniere's Disease?
  ➢ Episodic spinning vertigo, tinnitus, fullness sensation to affected ear, sensorineural hearing loss
790. What are the conservative treatment options?
  ➢ Low-sodium diet, diuretics, rest

## *Tinnitus*

791. What is tinnitus? What is it commonly associated with?

> ➤ Perception of noise (ringing, buzzing, pulsating)
> ➤ Sensorineural hearing loss

# Nose & Sinus Disorders

## *Epistaxis*

792. What are some treatment options for epistaxis?

> ➤ Direct pressure/clamping
> ➤ Topical – oxymetazoline, lidocaine, cocaine
> ➤ Silver nitrate/electrocautery
> ➤ Packing – if posterior, requires inpatient admission due to increased risk for hypoxia and cardiac arrhythmias
> ➤ Surgical intervention

793. If nasal packing is placed for epistaxis, when should it be removed?

> ➤ Within 24-48 hours

## *Allergic Rhinitis*

794. What are some signs and symptoms of allergic rhinitis?

> ➤ Ocular pruritis/watering, rhinorrhea, congestion, sneezing, allergic salute, allergic shiners, pale/boggy nasal mucosa, cobblestoning of the pharynx

795. What is the first line treatment for allergic rhinitis?

> ➤ Topical nasal steroid sprays daily

796. What is rhinitis medicamentosa?
  ➤ Rebound rhinorrhea associated with overuse of topic nasal decongestants (ie. neosynephrine or oxymetazoline)

## *Sinusitis*

797. What pathogens commonly cause acute sinusitis?
  ➤ Viral (most common) – adenovirus, rhinovirus, influenza, parainfluenza
  ➤ Bacterial – S. pneumoniae, H. flu, M. catarrhalis

798. What are risk factors for acute sinusitis?
  ➤ Recent URI
  ➤ Smoking
  ➤ Allergies
  ➤ History of facial trauma

799. What are the signs and symptoms of acute sinusitis?
  ➤ Fever, facial pain/pressure, purulent rhinorrhea, congestion, tenderness to palpation over sinuses with decreased transillumination

800. When should antibiotics be considered for acute sinusitis? What is the preferred antibiotic?
  ➤ Symptoms ≥10 days without improvement, onset with severe symptoms (purulent nasal discharge or facial pain)/high fever, or symptoms worsening after URI was beginning to improve
  ➤ Treatment – amoxicillin or amoxicillin-clavulanate x 7-10 days

801. What is chronic sinusitis? What is the treatment?

> Acute sinusitis that does not respond to treatment and lasts >12 weeks
> Treatment – amoxicillin-clavulanate x 21 days, intranasal glucocorticoids, saline irrigations, endoscopic sinus surgery

## Foreign Bodies

802. What is the common presentation of a nasal foreign body?
> Unilateral, foul-smelling rhinorrhea in a child
> Check all orifices

# Oropharyngeal Disorders

## Dental Abscess

803. What is the treatment for a patient with a dental abscess?
> Antibiotics – penicillin VK
> Incision and drainage (I&D)
> Urgent dental evaluation

804. What is the life-threatening, deep submandibular infection that occurs secondary to a dental infection called?
> Ludwig's Angina

## Vincent's Angina

805. What is Vincent's angina? How does it present?
> Necrotizing ulcerative gingivitis (aka "trench mouth")

> Gingival ulcerations, progressive painful infection, swelling and sloughing of dead tissue from the mouth

## Aphthous Ulcers

806. What is the common name for aphthous ulcers? How do they present?
> Canker sores
> Painful shallow ulcers with red halos and yellow-gray centers that occur on the oral mucosa

## Oral Candidiasis

807. What is the common name for oral candidiasis? What are some risk factors? How does it present?
> Thrush (not to be confused with leukoplakia)
> Immunocompromised (DM, HIV), antibiotic use, inhaled corticosteroid use
> White plaques on the oral mucosa that can be scraped off

808. What are the treatment options for oral candidiasis?
> Clotrimazole troches
> Nystatin rinses
> PO antifungals

## Leukoplakia

809. What is leukoplakia? How does it differ in appearance from oral candidiasis?
> Pre-malignant lesion of the oral mucosa

➢ White plaques cannot be scraped off (oral candidiasis can be scraped off)

## HSV-1

810. Which type of herpes typically occurs in or around the oral cavity? How does it present?
   ➢ Herpes simplex type 1 (HSV-1)
   ➢ Prodrome (fever, fatigue, tingling) followed by painful grouped vesicular lesions on erythematous base

## Laryngitis

811. What are the symptoms of laryngitis? What is the treatment?
   ➢ Hoarseness, cough
   ➢ Treatment – supportive treatment and vocal rest

## Peritonsillar Abscess

812. What are the signs and symptoms of a patient with a peritonsillar abscess (PTA)?
   ➢ Fever, sore throat, muffled "hot potato" voice, unilateral tonsillar swelling, uvula deviation, trismus

## Pharyngitis

813. What are common etiologies of pharyngitis?
   ➢ Viral (most common) – adenovirus, rhinovirus, coronavirus, parainfluenza, coxsackievirus, mononucleosis

> Bacterial – Group A beta-hemolytic streptococcus (GABHS)

814. What criteria is used to direct diagnosis and treatment of pharyngitis?

> CENTOR criteria
  - C: Cough absent
  - E: Exudate
  - N: Nodes
  - T: Temperature >38°C
  - OR: Young or old

815. What is the treatment for strep pharyngitis?

> PO penicillin or amoxicillin
> IM benzathine penicillin

816. What complications are associated with untreated strep pharyngitis? How do they present?

> Scarlet fever – fever, diffuse erythematous rash that blanches with "sandpaper-like" texture (desquamates), circumoral pallor, strawberry tongue
> Rheumatic fever – polyarthritis, carditis, subcutaneous nodules, erythema marginatum, Sydenham's chorea (Jones Criteria); can lead to chronic valvular disorders
> Do not miss epiglottitis if no exudates, severe throat pain or pain with wiggling thyroid gland

## *Sialadenitis*

817. What is sialadenitis? What are the treatment options?

➢ Inflammation and enlargement of the salivary glands
➢ **M**assage, **A**ntibiotics, **S**ialagogues, **H**ydration, Warm compresses
  ▪ Remember: "**MASH**"

818. What is a chronic autoimmune disorder that typically causes bilateral swelling of the parotid or submandibular glands, dry eyes, and dry mouth?
➢ Sjogren's Syndrome

## *Parotitis*

819. What condition is parotitis associated with? How does it present?
➢ Mumps
➢ Facial swelling (one or both salivary glands)

# 8

# GENITOURINARY
# SYSTEM

## *Incontinence*

### *General*

820. What is the smooth muscle of the bladder wall that contracts during urination to facilitate the release of urine?

> ➢ Detrusor muscle

821. What are the 5 types of urinary incontinence?

> ➢ Stress
> ➢ Urge
> ➢ Mixed
> ➢ Overflow
> ➢ Functional or transient

822. What type of nonpharmacologic treatment can be used to treat incontinence?

> ➢ Behavioral modifications, pessaries, pelvic floor training (ie. Kegels, PT)

### *Urge Incontinence*

823. What are the signs and symptoms of urge incontinence?

> ➢ Signs and symptoms of OAB + incontinence

824. What medications are used to treat OAB and urge incontinence?

> ➢ Anticholinergics – oxybutynin
> ➢ Beta-3 agonist – mirabegron

### *Stress Incontinence*

825. What is stress incontinence? What are the symptoms?

➤ Leakage of urine related to increased
intraabdominal pressure
  ▪ Most common form of incontinence in women
  ▪ Caused by pelvic floor and intrinsic sphincter
    disorder
➤ Incontinence with coughing, sneezing, laughing,
  exercising, lifting

## Mixed Incontinence

826. What is mixed incontinence?

➤ Urge incontinence + stress incontinence

## Overflow Incontinence

827. What are the most common causes for overflow
incontinence in men? In women? What is the
treatment?

➤ Men: BPH, urethral strictures
➤ Women: Cystocele
➤ Treatment: Surgical removal of obstruction,
  intermittent or indwelling catheterization

## Functional/Transient Incontinence

828. What are some causes for functional or transient
incontinence?

➤ UTI, delirium, medications, atrophic urethritis,
  vaginitis, psychologic, excess urinary output (ex.
  hyperglycemia, CHF), restricted mobility, stool
  impaction

## *Overactive Bladder*

829. What is the cause of overactive bladder (OAB)?
What are the signs and symptoms?
> Detrusor overactivity
> Signs/symptoms – frequency, urgency, nocturia

## *Infectious Disorders*

### *Cystitis*

830. What is acute cystitis?
> Inflammation/infection of the bladder

831. What organism is the most common cause of cystitis?
> Escherichia coli

832. What are classic clinical manifestations of cystitis?
> Dysuria, frequency, urgency, suprapubic pain
> Hematuria may also be present

833. What are the indications for treatment of asymptomatic bacteriuria?
> Pregnancy, urinary tract surgery/interventions

834. What UA abnormalities are suggestive of acute cystitis?
> Nitrites
> Leukocyte esterase
> Pyuria
> Bacteriuria

835. What laboratory test confirms acute cystitis?
> Urine culture

## *Pyelonephritis*

836. What is pyelonephritis?
> ➤ Inflammation/infection of the kidneys secondary to ascending lower urinary tract infection

837. What are signs and symptoms of pyelonephritis?
> ➤ Gradual onset dull, constant flank pain, fever, chills, nausea, vomiting
> ➤ CVA tenderness

838. What patients can be treated outpatient for pyelonephritis?
> ➤ Reassuring vital signs
> ➤ Can tolerate PO intake/antibiotic
> ➤ Can get antibiotic filled
> ➤ Not pregnant
> ➤ Not immunocompromised
> ➤ Those without significant comorbidities

## *Urethritis*

839. What organisms most commonly cause urethritis?
> ➤ Gonorrhea
> ➤ Chlamydia

## *Epididymitis*

840. What is epididymitis? What are the signs and symptoms?
> ➤ Inflammation/infection of the epididymis
> ➤ Fever, testicular pain/swelling

841. What is a normal cremasteric reflex?

> Elevation of the ipsilateral testes with stroking of the inner thigh

842. What is Prehn's sign?
> Elevation of the testes
  ▪ Positive – relief of pain
  ▪ Negative – no relief of pain

843. What physical exam findings support the diagnosis of epididymitis?
> Positive Prehn's sign
> Normal cremasteric reflex

## Orchitis

844. What is orchitis? What is it most commonly associated with?
> Inflammation/infection of the testes
> Mumps

## Prostatitis

845. What is prostatitis? What are the signs and symptoms of acute prostatitis?
> Inflammation/infection of the prostate
> Fever, chills, malaise, myalgia, dysuria, frequency, urgency, suprapubic/perineal pain, lower back pain

846. What are the most common pathogens involved in acute prostatitis?
> <35 years old – chlamydia, gonorrhea
> >35 years old – E. coli

847. What physical exam findings are suggestive of acute prostatitis?

➤ Digital rectal exam (DRE) – tender, boggy
prostate

848. Vigorous prostate exams should be avoided in
which type of prostatitis? Should also be avoided prior
to obtaining which lab test?

➤ Acute prostatitis

➤ PSA – may cause false elevation

849. What are some complications of acute bacterial
prostatitis?

➤ Prostatic abscess, epididymitis, chronic bacterial
prostatitis, bacteremia

### *Fournier Gangrene*

850. What necrotizing fasciitis of the perineum requires
immediate treatment and emergent surgical
consultation?

➤ Fournier gangrene

## *Neoplasms*
### *Bladder Cancer*

851. What is the most common presenting symptom
seen with bladder cancer?

➤ Intermittent, gross, painless hematuria

852. What test is considered the gold standard for the
initial diagnosis and staging of bladder cancer?

➤ Cystoscopy with biopsy

853. What is the greatest risk factor for bladder cancer?

➤ Smoking

### *Penile Cancer*

854. What is the most common form of penile cancer? What are the common clinical presentations?
> ➤ Squamous cell carcinoma (SCC)
> ➤ Painless penile lump or ulcer

### *Prostate Cancer*

855. What physical exam findings are worrisome for prostate cancer?
> ➤ Digital rectal exam – asymmetrically enlarged prostate with irregularities

856. What lab value is elevated in prostate cancer?
> ➤ PSA

857. What are other causes that can elevate PSA level?
> ➤ BPH, urinary retention, prostatitis

858. How is prostate cancer diagnosed?
> ➤ Prostate biopsy

### *Testicular Cancer*

859. What age group does testicular cancer typically present in?
> ➤ Young adult/middle-aged men

860. How does testicular cancer present?
> ➤ Painless mass on the testes

861. What hormone levels should be checked in a testicular mass? What is the next step in a patient who is found to have a solid testicular mass on ultrasonography?
> ➤ Hormones:
>   ▪ AFP

- LDH
- B-hCG
➢ Next step: Inguinal orchiectomy

## *Nephrolithiasis/Urolithiasis*

862. What are the types of kidney stones? Which is most common?
➢ Calcium oxalate (most common)
➢ Calcium phosphate
➢ Uric acid
➢ Struvite
➢ Cysteine

863. Where are the most common locations for a ureteral stone to become stuck?
➢ Ureterovesical junction (UVJ)
➢ Ureteropelvic junction (UPJ)
➢ At the level of the iliac vessels

864. What are signs and symptoms of nephrolithiasis/urolithiasis?
➢ Sudden onset sharp, colicky intermittent flank pain

865. What physical exam sign is associated with nephrolithiasis/urolithiasis? What urine abnormality may be seen?
➢ CVA tenderness
➢ Hematuria

866. What is the best test to evaluate for nephrolithiasis/urolithiasis?
➢ CT without contrast

867. What type of x-ray would show radiopaque kidney stones?

> KUB

868. Stones of what size typically will pass spontaneously? What size is unlikely to pass spontaneously?

> Spontaneously: ≤4 mm in diameter
> Unlikely to pass: ≥10 mm in diameter

869. What are the treatment options for nephrolithiasis/urolithiasis?

> Small (<10 mm) – fluids and analgesia, possible expulsion therapy
  ▪ May be removed surgically if obstructing or does not pass on its own
> Large (>10 mm) – fluids and analgesia, expulsion therapy or surgical intervention

870. What types are referred to as "infection stones" since they only form in the setting of UTIs?

> Struvite stones

871. When should hospitalization be considered for urolithiasis?

> Infected and obstructed stone, renal failure, single kidney, intractable pain, uncontrolled vomiting, renal transplant patient, failed outpatient medical therapy

## Urethral Disorders

872. What is the difference between urethra prolapse and stricture?

> Urethral prolapse – circumferential protrusion of the urethra through the external urethral opening
> Urethral stricture – narrowing of the urethra

## Penile Disorders

### Erectile Dysfunction

873. What is erectile dysfunction (ED)?
> Inability to achieve or maintain an erection

874. What are the treatment options for ED?
> Counseling
> Medications – vardenafil, tadalafil, sildenafil
> Injections/suppositories
> Vacuum devices
> Penile ring
> Implants/prostheses

### Epispadias/Hypospadias

875. What is the difference between epispadias and hypospadias in males?
> Epispadias – urethra is on dorsal side (top) of the penis
> Hypospadias – urethra is on ventral side (underside) of the penis

### Priapism

876. Which disease demographic is at increased risk of developing priapism?
> Males with sickle cell disease

877. What are some treatment options for priapism?

175

> Cavernosal blood aspiration
> Terbutaline
> Phenylephrine

## Peyronie's Disease

878. What disorder causes painful, curved penile erection due to the buildup of plaque in the corpus cavernousm?
> Peyronie's disease

## Phimosis/Paraphimosis

879. What is the difference between phimosis and paraphimosis?
> Phimosis – inability to retract the foreskin from the glans
  ▪ Can be a normal variant
  ▪ Painless
> Paraphimosis – inability to reduce the foreskin over the glans
  ▪ Emergency
  ▪ Painful

## Balanitis

880. What is balanitis? What are the risk factors? What are the signs and symptoms?
> Inflammation of the glans penis
> Risk factors - poor hygiene, uncircumcised, diabetes mellitus, immunocompromised, obesity

> Signs and symptoms - pain, tenderness, pruritus, erythema, exudate, or ulcerations of the glans and/or foreskin

881. What is the most common infection with balanitis?

> Candida

## Benign Prostatic Hyperplasia

882. What are classic symptoms associated with benign prostatic hyperplasia (BPH)?

> Hesitation, frequency, weak stream, incomplete emptying, postvoid dribbling, nocturia

883. What physical exam findings are suggestive of BPH?

> Digital rectal exam – symmetrically enlarged prostate

884. What are the treatment options for BPH?

> Medications – tamsulosin, finasteride
> Surgery – transurethral resection of prostate (TURP)
>  - Many alternative options are available

## Testicular Disorders

### Hydrocele/Varicocele

885. What is the difference between hydrocele and varicocele? What are the physical exam findings?

> Hydrocele – accumulation of fluid along the spermatic cord

- Physical exam – nontender fullness that transilluminates
➤ Varicocele – dilation of vessels within the spermatic cord
  - Physical exam – nontender mass that does not transilluminate, "bag of worms"

## *Testicular Torsion*

886. What is the classic presentation of testicular torsion?
➤ Unilateral testicular pain, lower abdominal pain, nausea, high riding testicle

887. What physical exam findings are worrisome for testicular torsion?
➤ Negative Prehn's sign
➤ Absent cremasteric reflex

888. What is the best test to confirm the diagnosis of testicular torsion?
➤ Testicular ultrasound with doppler

889. What is the definitive treatment for testicular torsion?
➤ Emergent surgical exploration with detorsion and orchiopexy

890. In what time should a torsed testicle be treated to provide the best viability?
➤ Detorsion within 4-6 hours

891. What are clinical findings for torsion of the appendix testis? In which age group is this most common?

> Nontender testicle; tender palpable polyp-like mass to the anterosuperior testicular surface
> "Blue dot sign"
  ▪ Subtle blue discoloration through the overlying skin due to infarction and necrosis of the appendix testis
> Common in school aged boys

## Cryptorchidism

892. What is cryptorchidism? What does it increase the risk of?
> Failure of one or both testes to descend
> Infertility and testicular cancer

# Genitourinary System

# 9

---

# REPRODUCTIVE SYSTEM

## *Breast Disorders*

893. What areas should be assessed during a breast examine for lymphadenopathy?

> Axillary, supraclavicular, infraclavicular regions

894. What is a cystic fluid collection of the breast that is usually caused by an obstructed milk duct?

> Galactocele

895. What is the most common benign breast tumor?

> Fibroadenomas

896. How do fibroadenomas typically present?

> Firm, smooth, painless, mobile breast masses that increase in size over several months

897. How does fibrocystic disease typically present?

> Breast pain, tenderness, and nodules that correlate with a woman's menstrual cycle

898. What is gynecomastia?

> Enlargement of breast tissue in males, sometimes uneven

899. What is the most common pathogen responsible for mastitis and breast abscesses in lactating women? What is the treatment?

> S. aureus

> Continued breastfeeding, antibiotics (dicloxacillin, oxacillin, nafcillin, cefalexin), aspiration/drainage if abscess present

900. What two laboratory studies should be obtained when physiologic bilateral milky nipple discharge is present?

> Prolactin and TSH levels

## Cervical Disorders

901. In general, what are the guidelines for cervical cancer screening? What procedure is used to biopsy the cervix after an abnormal Pap smear?

➤ Pap smear every 3 years from 21-65 years old
➤ Colposcopy

902. What is the most common abnormal Pap smear result?

➤ Atypical squamous cell of undetermined significance (ASC-US)

903. What are the treatment options for cervical dysplasia?

➤ Electrocautery
➤ Cryocautery
➤ Loop electrosurgical excision procedure (LEEP)
➤ Conization

## Complicated Pregnancy

904. What is the most common cause of spontaneous abortions/miscarriages? When do they most commonly occur?

➤ Chromosomal abnormalities
➤ First trimester

905. What are threatened, inevitable, incomplete, complete, and missed abortions?

➤ Threatened abortion – vaginal bleeding, viable intrauterine pregnancy, closed os
➤ Inevitable abortion – vaginal bleeding, viable intrauterine pregnancy, open os

> Incomplete abortion – vaginal bleeding, incomplete passage of products of conception, open os
> Complete abortion – vaginal bleeding, complete passage of products of conception, closed os
> Missed abortion – no vaginal bleeding, no passage of products of conception, closed os

906. What is abruptio placentae? What are the common risk factors? How does it present?

> Placental separation from the uterine wall prior to fetal delivery
> Trauma, drug use (cocaine), chronic vascular disorders
> Sudden, painful vaginal bleeding in a patient >20 weeks gestation

907. What is the treatment for abruptio placentae in pregnancy >23 weeks?

> Maternal resuscitation – blood products and coagulation factors
> Emergent C-section if signs of maternal or fetal distress
  ▪ Steroids if <37 weeks

908. What complication following C-section should be considered with the presentation of fever and uterine tenderness?

> Endometritis

909. What methods are used in the induction of labor?

> Laminaria
> Balloon catheter

> Intracervical prostaglandin gel or oral
> misoprostol

> IV oxytocin

910. What is an amniotomy?

> Manual rupture of membranes

911. What are the signs/symptoms of cord prolapse?
What is the treatment?

> Rope-like structure palpated on vaginal exam

> Immediate delivery

912. What is an ectopic pregnancy? What is the most
common location? What are the most common risk
factors?

> Implantation of fertilized ovum outside of the
> uterine cavity

> Ampulla of fallopian tube

> Pelvic inflammatory disease (PID), prior ectopic
> pregnancy, IUD, prior tubal procedures, and
> assisted reproductive techniques

913. How do ectopic pregnancies typically present?

> Adnexal pain/mass, amenorrhea, dizziness,
> syncope

914. How are ectopic pregnancies managed?

> Medical – methotrexate

> Surgical – laparoscopy or laparotomy

915. What is a heterotopic pregnancy?

> Presences of multiple pregnancies at two
> different implantation sites, usually an
> intrauterine and extrauterine pregnancy

916. When is screening for gestational diabetes
performed? What tests are used?

- 24-28 weeks gestation
- 1-hour 50 g non-fasting oral glucose tolerance test (OGTT)
  - Normal <140 mg/dL
    - If abnormal → 3-hour 100 g fasting oral glucose tolerance test (OGTT)

917. What is the first-line treatment for gestational diabetes? Second-line treatment?

- Diet, exercise, and close glucose monitoring
- Insulin if dietary treatment fails

918. What fetal complication is seen with gestational diabetes?

- Macrosomia

919. When in pregnancy ideally should a woman be screened for group B beta-hemolytic streptococcus (GBS) colonization? How are they screened?

- 36 weeks - 37 weeks and 6 days
- Both vaginal and rectal swabs

920. What is preeclampsia? What are the common signs/symptoms?

- Hypertension (>140/90) at >20 weeks gestation associated with end-organ damage
- Edema, visual disturbances, headaches

921. What laboratory abnormality is seen in patients with preeclampsia?

- Proteinuria

922. What is the most useful preventive pharmacologic intervention that can be taken to reduce the frequency of preeclampsia in pregnant women with moderate to high risk?

➤ Low-dose aspirin

923. What is the treatment for preeclampsia?

➤ Blood pressure control – labetalol, hydralazine, methyldopa, nifedipine

➤ Seizure prophylaxis – IV magnesium

924. What is eclampsia? How is it treated?

➤ Maternal seizures secondary to elevated blood pressure in the setting of preeclampsia

➤ Treatment – ABCs, seizure management, IV magnesium, prompt delivery of the infant

925. What is **HELLP** syndrome?

➤ Preeclampsia + **H**emolysis, **E**levated **L**iver enzymes, and **L**ow **P**latelet count

926. What is the treatment for incompetent cervix?

➤ Cervical cerclage

927. Why are steroids given before delivery in pregnancies <37 weeks?

➤ Promotes fetal lung maturity and surfactant production

928. What is placenta previa? What's the classic presentation?

➤ Placental tissue extending over the internal cervical os

➤ Painless vaginal bleeding in a patient >20 weeks gestation

929. What is the most common cause of postpartum hemorrhage? What are the treatment options?

➤ Uterine atony

> Fundal massage, medications (oxytocin, methylergonovine, misoprostol), blood products, surgery

930. What is premature rupture of membranes (PROM)? Premature preterm rupture of membranes (PPROM)?

> PROM – membrane rupture prior to the onset of labor
> PPROM – membrane rupture <37 weeks

931. What signs are suspicious for PROM/PPROM?

> Pooling of fluid
> Positive nitrazine paper test (blue)
> Ferning on microscopy

932. Which Rh factor in pregnancies requires administration of RhoGAM?

> Rh negative

933. What is shoulder dystocia? What is the sign associated with it? What is the first line treatment to correct it during delivery?

> Anterior shoulder becomes stuck behind the pubic symphysis during delivery
> Turtle sign – retraction of head
> McRoberts maneuver (hyperflexion of the mother's thighs toward the chest)
  ▪ Often used in conjunction with suprapubic pressure

## Contraceptive Methods

934. What are the most common complications associated with estrogen containing oral contraceptive

pills (OCPs) and estrogen hormone replacement
therapy (HRT)?

> DVT
> Hypertension
> Cardiovascular disease

935. What are the most common complications of
intrauterine devices (IUDs)?

> Ectopic pregnancy
> Infection/pelvic inflammatory disease (PID)
> Uterine perforation

## Menopause

936. How is menopause clinically diagnosed?

> Amenorrhea for 12 months in a woman >45
  years old without any other physiological or
  biologic causes

937. What are the common signs/symptoms of
menopause? What are the associated lab abnormalities?

> Spotting/cessation of menses, hot flashes,
  atrophic vaginitis, mood/sleep disturbances
> Low estrogen, high FSH (>30 mIU/mL)

## Menstrual Disorders

938. What is primary amenorrhea? Secondary
amenorrhea?

> Primary amenorrhea – absence of menstruation
  by 15 years old

> Secondary amenorrhea – absence of menses for three months in a woman who has previously menstruated

939. What are the stages of menstrual phases and when do they occur?

> Follicular phase: Begins at the start of menses & ends the day prior to the luteinizing hormone (LH) surge
> Luteal phase: Begins when LH surge occurs & ends at the start of the next menses

940. What is the first line non-hormonal pharmacologic therapy for primary dysmenorrhea?

> NSAIDs

941. What are the signs/symptoms of premenstrual syndrome (PMS)? When do they occur?

> Mood disturbances (anxiety, depression, emotional lability), fatigue, changes in appetite/sleep patterns, fluid retention (bloating, edema, breast tenderness)
> Begin during the luteal phase (1-2 weeks before menses) and end near the beginning of menses

942. What is dysfunctional uterine bleeding?

> Uterine bleeding in the absence of anatomical abnormalities

943. What is Mittelschmerz?

> Pelvic pain that occurs mid-cycle
    ▪ Secondary to ovarian follicle rupture

## *Neoplasms*

944. What is the most common presenting symptom of endometrial cancer? What is the gold standard for diagnosis?

> ➤ Postmenopausal bleeding
> ➤ Endometrial biopsy

945. What signs/symptoms are associated with ovarian cancer?

> ➤ Abdominal bloating, abdominal distention, pelvic pain, changes in bowel habits, lower back pain, urinary urgency/frequency

946. What tumor marker is associated with ovarian cancer?

> ➤ CA-125

947. Which strains of HPV are considered high-risk because they are associated with the development of cervical dysplasia/carcinoma? What vaccination offers protection against HPV?

> ➤ 16 and 18
> ➤ Gardasil

948. How does vulvar cancer typically present?

> ➤ Pruritic vulvar lesion

949. What is the most common type of breast cancer? What is the most common location on the breast?

> ➤ Invasive ductal carcinoma
> ➤ Upper outer quadrant

950. What physical exam findings are concerning for breast cancer?

> ➤ Irregular shaped, immobile, painless mass

➤ Skin changes (peau d'orange), clear-bloody nipple discharge, nipple retraction, dimpling of skin

951. Which breast disease causes chronic scaly, eczematous type rash that involves the nipple and areola? What type of breast cancer is it associated with?

➤ Paget disease of the breast

➤ Ductal carcinoma in situ (DCIS)

952. What screening test is used to evaluate for breast carcinoma? How is it definitively diagnosed?

➤ Mammogram

➤ Core needle biopsy or FNA biopsy

953. What is the area of breast tissue that extends laterally toward the axilla called?

➤ Tail of Spence

954. What are the indications of genetic testing for BRCA mutation?

➤ Any of the following:
  ▪ Triple negative breast cancer ≤60 years old
  ▪ Male breast cancer
  ▪ Breast cancer at any age and a relative with breast cancer diagnosed ≤50 years old
  ▪ Breast cancer diagnosis ≤45 years old

## Ovarian Disorders

955. What are differential diagnoses for ruptured ovarian cyst?

➤ Ectopic pregnancy, appendicitis, PID, tubo-ovarian abscess

956. What are the signs/symptoms of polycystic ovary syndrome (PCOS)? What is seen on pelvic ultrasound?

> Amenorrhea/oligomenorrhea, infertility, obesity, hirsutism, acne, insulin resistance
> "String of pearls" on ovaries

957. What is the classic presentation of ovarian torsion? What is the best imaging modality? How is it treated?

> Acute onset lower pelvic pain, nausea, vomiting, adnexal tenderness
> Transvaginal ultrasound with doppler
> Urgent laparoscopy

## Sexually Transmitted Infections & Pelvic Inflammatory Disease

958. Which two sexually transmitted infections (STIs) can present asymptomatically or with vaginitis, urethritis, cervicitis, salpingitis, and are cotreated together? What are the 2021 CDC recommendations for treatment?

> Gonorrhea – ceftriaxone 500mg IM once
> Chlamydia – doxycycline 100mg PO BID x 7 days (or in pregnant women azithromycin 1g single dose therapy)

959. What are the classic signs and symptoms associated with Trichomonas? What is seen microscopically? How is it treated?

> Malodorous, yellow/green discharge, "strawberry cervix"
> Flagellated trichomonads

➤ Treatment – PO metronidazole

960. What are the most common organisms associated with the development of Pelvic Inflammatory Disease (PID)? What are the clinical signs and symptoms? What is the treatment?

➤ Chlamydia and gonorrhea

➤ Fever, mucopurulent cervical discharge, uterine/adnexal tenderness, cervical motion tenderness (CMT) on bimanual exam ("chandelier sign")

➤ Antibiotics (ceftriaxone and doxycycline), possible surgical intervention

961. What are the complications of chronic PID?

➤ Perihepatitis, ectopic pregnancy, tubo-ovarian abscess

962. Which type of herpes typically occurs on the genitalia? How does it present?

➤ Herpes simplex type 2 (HSV-2)

➤ Prodrome (fever, fatigue, tingling) followed by painful grouped vesicular lesions on an erythematous base

963. Which strains of HPV are associated with the development of condyloma acuminate (genital warts)? How do they present?

➤ 6 and 11

➤ Flesh-colored, "cauliflower-like" lesions on the genitalia

## *Trauma*

964. What testing/treatment should be offered after sexual assault?
> - Beta-hCG +/- emergency contraception
> - STI testing/cultures +/- post-exposure prophylaxis (PEP)
> - +/- tetanus booster
> - SANE exam
> - Counseling, consult local SART team, and follow-up

965. What are red flags or warning signs that a patient may be a victim of human trafficking?
> - Hesitancy in answering questions regarding injuries, inconsistent or scripted history, fearfulness or nervous behavior and demeanor, unawareness of current location
> - Multiple pregnancies, miscarriages, and recurrent or untreated sexually transmitted infections

966. During resuscitation of a pregnant patient, what can be performed to decrease compression on the inferior vena cava by the gravid uterus?
> - Manual left uterine displacement

## *Uncomplicated Pregnancy*

967. What are the signs and symptoms associated with pregnancy?
> - Amenorrhea, nausea/vomiting, breast tenderness/swelling, fatigue, urinary frequency/nocturia, melasma, linea nigra

> Chadwick sign – blue/violet discoloration of the cervix/vagina
> Goodell sign – softening of the cervix
> Hegar sign – softening of uterus

968. What shorthand method is used to report a woman's reproductive history?

> **GP** or **GTPAL**
  - **G**ravida (pregnancies)
  - **P**ara (deliveries)
  - **T**erm births
  - **P**reterm births (<37 weeks)
  - **A**bortions
  - **L**iving children

969. Which ultrasound findings confirm an intrauterine pregnancy?

> Intrauterine yolk sac OR an intrauterine fetus
  - Note: Presence of a gestational sac does not confirm an IUP

970. When can a yolk sac and fetal cardiac activity be visualized on ultrasound?

> Yolk sac – 5 weeks gestation
> Fetal cardiac activity – 5-6 weeks gestation

971. By how much should beta-hCG rise in an early, viable pregnancy?

> Doubles every 48 hours

972. What is a normal fetal heart rate?

> 110-160 bpm

973. Where should the uterine fundus be palpable at 12 weeks gestation? 20 weeks? >20 weeks?

> 12 weeks – pubic symphysis

- ➤ 20 weeks – umbilicus
- ➤ >20 weeks – distance in cm from pubic symphysis to fundus = weeks gestation

974. When during pregnancy should a woman receive a Tdap vaccine? Why?

- ➤ 3rd Trimester
- ➤ Protects against pertussis

975. What are the stages of labor?

- ➤ First stage – onset of contractions through full cervical dilation (10 cm)
- ➤ Second stage – full cervical dilation through delivery of the infant
- ➤ Third stage – delivery of the infant through delivery of the placenta
- ➤ Fourth stage – recovery (treatment of lacerations, tears, hemorrhage)

976. What are the components of the **APGAR** score? When is it assessed? How is it scored?

- ➤ **A**ppearance, **P**ulse, **G**rimace, **A**ctivity, **R**espirations
- ➤ 1, 5, and 10 minutes (if needed)
- ➤ 0-2 points for each category, max of 10 (higher score is desirable)

977. What structures are present in the umbilical cord?

- ➤ 2 arteries and 1 vein

978. How long does the postpartum period last? What should be addressed at the first visit after delivery?

- ➤ 6 weeks after delivery
- ➤ Postpartum depression, lactation, lochia, and birth control

979. What antihypertensive medications are absolute contraindications during pregnancy?

> Angiotensin receptor blocker (ARBs) and angiotensin converting enzyme inhibitors (ACEi)

## Uterine Disorders

980. What is endometriosis? What are the classic signs and symptoms? How is it diagnosed?

> Endometrial tissue located outside of the uterus
> Dysmenorrhea, dyspareunia, dyschezia
> Direct visualization on laparoscopy

981. What are considered first-line treatment options for endometriosis?

> NSAIDs
> Estrogen-progestin contraceptives

982. What is the common name for leiomyoma? What are the common signs and symptoms?

> Uterine fibroid
> Abnormal vaginal bleeding and palpable uterine mass

## Vaginal & Vulvar Disorders

983. What are the signs and symptoms of candidal vaginitis? What is seen on wet prep with KOH? What is the treatment?

> Thick, white, "cottage cheese-like" vaginal discharge, pruritis
> Pseudohyphae and/or hyphae with budding yeast

> Treatment – topical or PO antifungals

984. What causes atrophic vaginitis? What are the treatment options?

> Decrease in estrogen in postmenopausal women
> Treatment – vaginal lubricants, topical estrogen, hormone replacement therapy (HRT)

985. How does bacterial vaginosis (BV) present? What is noted on microscopy? What test is positive with the addition of KOH? What is the treatment?

> Thin, grey-white vaginal discharge with "fishy" odor
> Clue cells, positive whiff test
  - Treatment – topical or PO metronidazole

986. What is the most common treatment for a Bartholin cyst or abscess?

> Incision & drainage

987. What is the most common symptom associated with lichen sclerosis? What test confirms the diagnosis? What is the first-line medication treatment?

> Vulvar pruritus
> Tissue biopsy
> Topical corticosteroids

## Miscellaneous

988. What is the five staging system used to categorize sexual maturity from prepuberty to adult development? What development features does the staging system consist of?

> Tanner stages
> Pubic hair, breast development, genital changes

199

989. What is a common cause of an erythematous pruritic rash underneath the breast of a woman? What is the treatment?

> ➤ Cutaneous candidiasis
> ➤ Nystatin cream or powder

**10**

# NEUROLOGIC
# SYSTEM

# Headaches

## Migraines

990. What is the classic presentation of a migraine headache?

> Unilateral throbbing/pulsating pain with associated photophobia/phonophobia, nausea, vomiting +/- aura (transient visual/neurologic disturbances)

991. What are some triggers associated with migraine headaches?

> Menstruation, increased stress, nitrates, wine/alcohol, weather changes, change or irregular of sleep pattern, fasting, dehydration

992. What are some nonpharmacologic options for managing migraine headaches?

> Avoid headache triggers, healthy diet, regular exercise, decrease stress levels, regular sleep pattern, avoid excessive alcohol, avoid excessive caffeine, exercise regularly, hydration

993. What is first line treatment for a mild to moderate migraine? What treatment may be indicated if there is no response to first line medications?

> First line: Aspirin, NSAIDs, or Tylenol
> Triptan

994. What medications can be considered for migraine prophylaxis?

> Tricyclic antidepressants
> Beta blockers
> Valproic acid
> Topiramate

➤ Venlafaxine
➤ Botox
➤ Calcitonin gene-related peptide receptor (CGRP) antagonists
  ▪ Newer medication, but strong data to support utility in migraine prophylaxis

## Cluster Headaches

995. What are the classic characteristics of a cluster headache?
➤ Severe unilateral or periorbital headache lasting minutes to hours
➤ Unilateral tearing, nasal congestion, or rhinorrhea
➤ Ptosis or miosis

996. What is the treatment for acute cluster headaches? What can be used for prophylaxis?
➤ Acute treatment: Triptan (typically subcutaneous or intranasal) or oxygen
➤ Prophylaxis: Verapamil

## Tension Headaches

997. What is the classic presentation of a tension headache?
➤ Generalized/band-like pain

998. What nonpharmacological techniques are used to manage tension headaches? What medication may be used to prevent chronic tension headaches?
➤ Relaxation techniques
➤ Acetaminophen, aspirin, or NSAIDs

## _Trigeminal Neuralgia_

999. What are the signs and symptoms of trigeminal neuralgia?

> Episodic, unilateral electric shock-like pain that shoots from mouth to ear and is triggered by touch, eating, talking, and cold drafts

1000. What medications are used in the treatment of trigeminal neuralgia?

> Carbamazepine
> Oxcarbamazepine

## _Idiopathic Intracranial Hypertension_

1001. What is another name of idiopathic intracranial hypertension (IIH)?

> Pseudotumor cerebri

1002. What are classic clinical presentations/risk factors for idiopathic intracranial hypertension?

> Female of childbearing age
> Overweight
> Complains of headaches
> Papilledema seen on funduscopic exam

## _Red Flag Symptoms_

1003. What are the red flag symptoms for headaches that could indicate the presence of a serious underlying disorder?

> **S**ystemic symptoms: Fever, neoplasm, HIV, immunocompromised
> **N**eurologic symptoms: AMS, decreased consciousness, seizure

> **O**nset: Sudden or abrupt
> **O**lder patient: >50 years old with new onset
> **P**revious headache history: Onset of new headache, pattern change
> **P**regnancy or postpartum
>   - Remember: "**<u>SNOOP2</u>**"

## *Closed Head Injuries*

1004. What are the symptoms of a concussion?

> Amnesia, confusion, irritability, difficulty concentrating, headache, nausea, vomiting, dizziness

1005. What is the name for the condition in which concussion symptoms persist beyond the normal timeframe of recovery (weeks to months)?

> Post-concussion syndrome

1006. What are concerning findings on physical exam for an infant presenting with a head injury?

> Altered mental status (GCS ≤14)
> Palpable or depressed skull fracture
> Scalp hematoma
> Bulging anterior fontanelle
> Signs of basilar skull fracture
> Increased head circumference

1007. What are signs of basilar skull fracture?

> Periorbital ecchymosis (Raccoon eyes)
> Posterior auricular ecchymosis (Battle sign)
> Hemotympanum
> CSF otorrhea or rhinorrhea

205

1008. What is the decision-making scoring tool used to help predict if brain imaging is indicated for a pediatric head injury with GCS of ≤ 14?

> PECARN rules

1009. What is the decision-making tool used to clear adults with head injuries without obtaining CT head imaging?

> Canadian Head CT Rule

## Cranial Nerve Palsies

1010. What are the cranial nerves and their major functions? Which are motor? Sensory? Both?

> CN I – olfactory (sensory)
  - Smell
> CN II – optic (sensory)
  - Vision
> CN III – oculomotor (motor)
  - Extraocular muscles (EOMs)
    • Superior rectus, inferior rectus, medial rectus and inferior oblique muscles
  - Pupillary dilation/constriction
> CN IV – trochlear (motor)
  - EOM – superior oblique muscle
> CN V – trigeminal (sensory and motor)
  - 3 branches – ophthalmic, maxillary, mandibular
  - Mastication
> CN VI – abducens (motor)
  - EOM – lateral rectus muscle

- CN VII – facial (sensory and motor)
  - Facial expressions
  - Anterior 2/3rd tongue
- CN VIII – vestibulocochlear (sensory)
  - Hearing
  - Balance
- CN IX – glossopharyngeal (sensory and motor)
  - Swallowing, talking, gag reflex
  - Regulation of heart rate (via carotid receptors)
  - Posterior 1/3rd tongue
- CN X – vagus (sensory and motor)
  - Swallowing, talking, gag reflex
  - Regulation of heart rate, respiration, and digestion
  - Uvula/soft palate
- CN XI – accessory (motor)
  - Sternocleidomastoid (SCM) and trapezius muscles
- CN XII – hypoglossal (motor)
  - Tongue movement

## *Encephalopathic Disorders*

### *Encephalopathy*

1011. What are the signs and symptoms of encephalopathy?

- AMS, confusion, agitation, disturbed sleep-wake cycles, hallucinations, stupor, coma

1012. What physical exam finding is suggestive of hepatic encephalopathy? What lab abnormality is associated with this diagnosis? What are the treatment options?

➤ Asterixis

➤ Lab abnormality – elevated ammonia

➤ Treatment – lactulose, rifaximin

1013. What causes Wernicke encephalopathy? What is a common risk factor?

➤ Thiamine (vitamin B1) deficiency

➤ Alcohol abuse

1014. What is the classic triad of Wernicke encephalopathy?

➤ Encephalopathy (AMS), oculomotor dysfunction (nystagmus), ataxia

1015. What is the treatment for Wernicke encephalopathy?

➤ IV thiamine

➤ IV glucose

1016. If left untreated, what does Wernicke encephalopathy lead to?

➤ Wernicke-Korsakoff syndrome – permanent brain damage and short-term memory loss

## Reye Syndrome

1017. Which rare syndrome is primarily seen in children after a viral illness that may cause encephalopathy with hepatic dysfunction?

➤ Reye Syndrome

1018. What medication, if administrated to children, is considered a risk factor for development of Reye syndrome?

➤ Aspirin

## Infectious Disorders

### *Encephalitis & Meningitis*

1019. What is the difference between encephalitis and meningitis?

➤ Encephalitis – inflammation/infection of the brain parenchyma

➤ Meningitis – inflammation/infection of the dura

1020. What is the most common overall cause of encephalitis?

➤ HSV-1

1021. What are the most common organisms that cause bacterial meningitis?

➤ S. pneumoniae

➤ N. meningitidis

➤ Listeria (very young, very old, immunocompromised)

➤ Group B step (neonates)

➤ E. coli (neonates)

1022. What is the classic triad of meningitis?

➤ Fever, headache, nuchal rigidity

1023. What are two physical exam test that are used to evaluate for suspected meningitis?

➤ Kernig's sign – pain/stiffness of hamstring limits straightening leg when the hip is flexed

➤ Brudzinski's sign – passive flexion of the neck results in hip flexion

1024. What test must be ordered to differentiate between bacterial and viral meningitis?

> Lumbar puncture (LP) with cerebrospinal fluid (CSF) analysis

1025. What test should be ordered prior to an LP if a patient has papilledema?

> CT

1026. What would CSF analysis show in a patient with bacterial meningitis?

> Elevated WBC
  - Predominantly neutrophils
> Elevated protein
> Decreased glucose

1027. What would CSF analysis show in a patient with viral meningitis?

> Elevated WBC – predominantly lymphocytes
> Normal protein
> Normal glucose

1028. What antibiotic regimen is used for empiric treatment of meningitis?

> Ceftriaxone and vancomycin
  - Add ampicillin in patients ≥50 years old

1029. What are contraindications to a lumbar puncture?

> Space occupying lesion (ie. brain mass, abscess), cerebral edema, or obstructive hydrocephalus seen on CT imaging
> Skin infection or cellulitis at the puncture site
> Bleeding disorder, thrombocytopenia, on anticoagulation therapy
> Congenital spine abnormalities

1030. What are treatment options for post-dural puncture headache?

➢ Bedrest, oral analgesics, PO/IV rehydration, epidural blood patch

# Movement Disorders

## Essential Tremors

1031. Benign essential tremor improves with the ingestion of what substance?
➢ Alcohol

## Huntington Disease

1032. What are the signs and symptoms of Huntington disease?
➢ Chorea, dementia, behavioral changes (agitation, irritability)

## Parkinson Disease

1033. What are the classic signs and symptoms of Parkinson disease?
➢ Resting "pill-rolling" tremor, cogwheel rigidity, bradykinesia, postural instability, wide-based gait

1034. What is first line medication for Parkinson's disease?
➢ Levodopa combined with carbidopa

# Neurocognitive Disorders

## Delirium, Dementia, & Alzheimer's Disease

1035. What are the major differences between the presentation of delirium and dementia?
➢ Delirium – onset over hours to days, altered level of consciousness, agitation, restlessness

> Dementia – gradual onset over months to years, alert with impaired cognition, progressive course

1036. What is the treatment for delirium?

> Reorientation
> Elimination of precipitating factors
> Antipsychotics
  - Only used for hyperactive delirium when safety is a concern

1037. What are the differences in presentation between Alzheimer's disease and vascular dementia?

> Alzheimer's disease – gradual, progressive decline
> Vascular dementia – stepwise decline, neurovascular disease

1038. What should elderly patients with increasing memory loss and decreased functional status be screened for?

> Depression
> Vitamin B12 deficiency
> Hypothyroidism
> Tertiary syphilis

1039. What medications are used in the treatment of Alzheimer's disease?

> Acetylcholinesterase inhibitors – donepezil
> NMDA receptor antagonists – memantine

1040. What form of dementia is characterized by early and prominent behavioral changes?

> Frontotemporal dementia

1041. What disorder is frontotemporal dementia associated with?

➤ Amyotrophic lateral sclerosis (ALS)

1042. What form of dementia is characterized by mild Parkinsonism and visual hallucinations?

➤ Dementia with Lewy bodies

# Neuromuscular Disorders

## Cerebral Palsy

1043. What is cerebral palsy?

➤ Nonprogressive upper motor neuron disease that occurs following injury to the developing brain

## Multiple Sclerosis

1044. How does multiple sclerosis (MS) most commonly present?

➤ Visual disturbances (optic neuritis) and neurologic symptoms in a young adult/middle aged female

1045. What tests are used to diagnose MS?

➤ CSF analysis – elevated IgG, oligoclonal bands
➤ MRI – demyelinating lesions
➤ Evoked potentials (how long for a nerve/part of the brain to respond to stimulation)

1046. What is the treatment for a MS flare?

➤ IV steroids
  ▪ As long as there is no underlying infection

## Myasthenia Gravis

1047. What is myasthenia gravis?

➤ Autoimmune destruction of acetylcholine receptors

1048. What are the classic symptoms of myasthenia gravis?

➤ Proximal muscle weakness (worse with exertion/improves with rest), ptosis, diplopia, dysconjugate gaze

1049. What are the initial treatment options for myasthenia gravis?

➤ Pyridostigmine/neostigmine
➤ Immunosuppressants/corticosteroids (no steroids in myasthenic crisis)

## ALS (Lou Gehrig's Disease)

1050. What is another name for ALS?

➤ Lou Gehrig's disease

1051. What is the classic presentation of ALS?

➤ Muscle weakness/stiffness/cramping, postural instability, cognitive impairment (frontotemporal dementia)

# Peripheral Nerve Disorders
## Carpal Tunnel Syndrome

1052. What nerve is involved in carpal tunnel syndrome? What are two exam maneuvers used to assess for it?

➤ Median nerve
➤ Tinel's and Phalen's test

1053. What diagnostic tools can be used to support clinical suspension for the diagnosis of carpal tunnel syndrome?

> Nerve conduction studies (NCS)
> Electromyography (EMG)

1054. What are some treatment options of carpal tunnel syndrome?

> Activity modifications
> Night splinting
> Corticosteroids
> Surgical intervention

### *Guillain-Barre Syndrome*

1055. What is Guillain-Barre Syndrome (GBS)?

> Inflammatory peripheral neuropathy that occurs after a URI or GI illness (campylobacter), vaccinations, or procedures/medication administration

1056. What are the classic symptoms of GBS?

> Symmetrical ascending weakness/paralysis and loss of DTRs

1057. What findings are seen on CSF analysis in patient with GBS?

> Elevated protein with normal cell counts

1058. What is the treatment for GBS?

> IVIG or plasmapheresis
> Supportive care – intubation if respiratory involvement

## *Diabetic Neuropathy*

1059. What is the distribution of peripheral neuropathy seen in patients with diabetes mellitus?

➤ "Stocking and glove"

## *Bell's Palsy*

1060. What is Bell's palsy?

➤ Unilateral palsy of CN VII (facial nerve)

1061. How can you differentiate between a Bell's palsy and a stroke on physical exam?

➤ Bell's palsy – loss of muscle tone over forehead (cannot raise eyebrows and wrinkle forehead)

➤ Stroke – forehead muscles are spared (can raise eyebrows and wrinkle forehead)

1062. What are the common signs and symptoms of Bell's palsy?

➤ Unilateral facial droop (involving the forehead), ptosis, decreased tear production, decreased salivation, altered taste, tinnitus, hyperacusis

1063. What is the treatment for Bell's palsy?

➤ Corticosteroids

➤ Eye patch and lubricating eye drops

➤ Antiviral medications – if concerned for herpes zoster

➤ Doxycycline if concerned for Lyme disease

## *Seizure Disorders*

### *General*

1064. What is the difference between focal and generalized seizures?
  - Focal: Seizures arise from a discrete area of the cerebral cortex
  - Generalized: Seizures arise from both hemispheres of the brain simultaneously

1065. What is the classic presentation associated with a simple focal seizure?
  - Jacksonian march

1066. What are two other names used to describe a generalized convulsive seizure?
  - Grand mal seizure
  - Tonic-clonic seizure

1067. What is the postictal phase?
  - Period after seizure but before patient wakes up
    - Begins when twitching movements stop, usually deep sleep & deep breathing occurs, may have confusion or agitation

1068. What type of seizure is typically associated with incontinence, tongue and/or cheek biting?
  - Tonic-clonic

1069. What is an essential diagnostic tool used to help assess for abnormal brainwaves and support diagnosis of epileptic seizures?
  - Electroencephalography (EEG)

1070. What other studies that may be ordered for new onset seizures in adults?
  - Electrolytes (glucose, calcium, magnesium)

> CBC
> Renal function tests
> Liver function test
> Urinalysis, urine pregnancy test
> Toxicology screening
> Lactic acid
> Electrocardiogram (ECG) to assess QT interval
> Lumbar puncture
> MRI or CT scan

1071. What are some examples of anti-convulsant medications used in the treatment of seizures?

> Phenytoin
> VPA/Depakote
> Topiramate
> Lamotrigine
> Carbamazepine
> Oxcarbamazepine
> Levetiracetam
> Ethosuximide
> Benzodiazepines for acute seizure

## Absence Seizures

1072. How do absence seizures present?

> Brief period of "spacing-out" associated with motor activity (ie. blinking, chewing, twitching)

## Febrile Seizures

1073. What is the most common age for simple febrile seizures in children?

> 6 months to 5 years old

1074. How do simple febrile seizures usually present?

➤ Generalized seizure, last < 15 minutes, occur once in a 24-hour period, no focal findings

➤ Fever (rapid increase in temperature occurs)

➤ Usually with associated viral or bacterial infection

### Status Epilepticus

1075. How is status epilepticus defined?

➤ Seizure activity ≥5 minutes without a return to baseline

➤ ≥2 recurrent seizures without full recovery of consciousness between seizures

1076. What is the first line treatment for status epilepticus?

➤ Benzodiazepines – lorazepam or diazepam

## Vascular Disorders
### Cerebral Aneurysms & Hemorrhage

1077. What is the most common type of cerebral aneurysm? Where is it most commonly located?

➤ Berry (saccular) aneurysm

➤ Circle of Willis

1078. How does an epidural hematoma typically present?

➤ Loss of consciousness → lucid interval → sudden deterioration

1079. How does an epidural hematoma appear on a CT of the head?

➢ Lens shaped

1080. What are some risk factors for developing a subdural hematoma? What artery is most commonly involved?

➢ Risk factors – alcohol abuse, advanced age, anticoagulant use
➢ Middle meningeal artery

1081. How does a subdural hematoma appear on a CT of the head?

➢ Crescent shaped

1082. What condition predisposes a patient to intracerebral hemorrhage?

➢ Hypertension

1083. What conditions predispose a patient to SAH? What is the most common cause of SAH?

➢ Cerebral aneurysms – Berry (saccular) aneurysms
➢ AV malformations
➢ Most common cause – trauma

1084. How does non-traumatic SAH present?

➢ Sudden onset, "thunderclap" headache with or without exertional activity (sex/intercourse, exercise)

1085. What may be seen on CSF analysis in a with SAH?

➢ RBCs in all 4 tubes
➢ Xanthochromia

## Stroke & TIA

1086. What are the two main types of strokes? Which is the most common?

➢ Ischemic (most common)

➢ Hemorrhagic

1087. What are the types of ischemic strokes? Which is the most common? What is the most common modifiable cause of ischemic stroke?

➢ Thrombotic (most common)

➢ Embolic

➢ Systemic hypoperfusion

➢ Modifiable cause – hypertension

1088. What major signs and symptoms are seen in a patient with an anterior, middle, or posterior cerebral artery stroke?

➢ Anterior cerebral artery – contralateral leg weakness > arm weakness

➢ Middle cerebral artery – contralateral arm > leg weakness/paresthesias, facial droop, aphasia, homonymous hemianopsia, unilateral neglect

➢ Posterior cerebral artery – contralateral visual field deficits, dizziness

1089. What major signs and symptoms are seen a patient with a cerebellar stroke?

➢ Ataxia and impaired coordination – difficulty with heel to shin test, rapid alternating movements, and finger to nose test, positive pronator drift and Romberg tests

1090. What tests should be done in all patients with a TIA or stroke?

➢ CT head without contrast

➢ ECG and telemetry

➢ Cerebrovascular imaging (head and neck vessels)

> Echocardiogram
> Hemoglobin A1c and lipid panel

1091. What is the time window for administration of tissue plasminogen activator (tPA) for ischemic strokes?

> Within 4.5 hours

1092. What are the exclusion criteria for tPA administration?

> Absolute contraindications:
  - Intracranial or systemic hemorrhage
  - SBP >185 or DBP >110 mmHg
> Relative contraindications:
  - Current use of anticoagulation
  - Increased risk of bleeding (ie. recent ischemic stroke, significant GI bleeding history, coagulopathic)

1093. What are the two main types of hemorrhagic strokes? Which is the most common?

> Intracerebral hemorrhage (most common)
> Subarachnoid hemorrhage (SAH)

1094. What is the difference between decorticate and decerebrate posturing? Which is more worrisome?

> Decorticate – flexed arms, hands drawn in toward the "core"
> Decerebrate – extended arms/legs, arched neck/back (indicative of more severe brain damage)

1095. What is a transient ischemic attack (TIA)?

> Neurological deficit that completely resolves within 24 hours

1096. What initial tests may be used to assess for carotid etiology of a TIA? If carotid stenosis is present, what is the surgical treatment?
> Carotid ultrasound or CT Angiogram
> Treatment – carotid endarterectomy (CEA)

## *Giant Cell Arteritis (GCA)*

1097. What other disease is commonly associated with GCA?
> Polymyalgia rheumatica (PMR)

1098. What are the common symptoms of GCA?
> Unilateral temporal headache, jaw claudication, scalp tenderness, tender/enlarged temporal artery

1099. What lab marker will be elevated in a patient with GCA?
> ESR >50

1100. How is GCA diagnosed?
> Temporal artery biopsy

1101. What is the treatment for GCA?
> High dose corticosteroids

1102. If GCA is left untreated, what complication may occur?
> Blindness

# *Miscellaneous*

## *Reflexes*

1103. What are the four major deep tendon reflexes, and what are the associated nerve roots?
> Biceps (C5, C6)

> Triceps (C7)
> Patellar (L3, L4)
> Achilles (S1)

1104. What is the grading scale for assessing reflexes? Which reflex gradings are considered abnormal?

> 0 (absent)
> +1 (diminished)
> +2 (normal)
> +3 (brisk)
> +4 (hyperactive, non-sustained clonus)
> +5 (sustained clonus)
  - Abnormal: 0, +4, +5

1105. What can a sunken or depressed anterior fontanelle suggest?

> Dehydration or malnutrition

1106. What can a tense or bulging fontanelle suggest? What are some diagnoses that can cause this physical exam finding?

> Increased intracranial pressure
> Subdural hematoma or meningitis

1107. When does the Moro reflex in infants normally disappear by?

> 3-6 months of age

1108. What clinical features of fetal alcohol syndrome (FAS)?

> Microcephaly
> Short palpebral fissures (narrow eyes)
> Thin vermillion border and smooth philtrum
> Flat nasal bridge

1109. What are risk factors associated with Sudden Infant Death Syndrome (SIDS)?

> Prematurity, low birth weight, prone sleeping position, bed sharing, maternal smoking, overheating, sleeping on a soft surface or with loose blankets/pillows

## Neoplasms

1110. What is the most common type of brain neoplasm?

> Metastatic lesion

1111. What are the three most common malignancies that metastasize to the brain?

> Breast
> Lung
> Melanoma

1112. How is a test of skew performed? What does a positive test of shew suggest?

> Examiner covers one of the patient's eye, then when eye is uncovered assesses for a vertical shift in the eye
> Brainstem or cerebellar lesion

## Vertigo

1113. What are the three tests performed in the HINTS examination? If the HINTS examination is positive, what does it suggest?

> Head impulse test, assessment for direction-changing nystagmus, and a test of skew
> Central vertigo rather than peripheral vertigo

1114. What is considered a positive Romberg test?

> Patient sways (versus becomes markedly more unsteady) when standing upright with feet together and eyes closed

## *Abuse*

1115. What should infants who are diagnosed with subdural hematoma or subarachnoid hemorrhage also be evaluated for?

> Physical abuse

1116. What abnormal eye exam finding is commonly seen with abusive head trauma in children?

> Retinal hemorrhages

# 11

## HEMATOLOGIC SYSTEM

## *Idiopathic Thrombocytopenic Purpura*

1117. What is Idiopathic Thrombocytopenic Purpura (ITP)? How does it present? What are the treatment options?

> ➤ Autoimmune dysfunction resulting in destruction of platelets and isolated thrombocytopenia
>   - Often caused by a viral infection
> ➤ Petechiae/purpura, epistaxis, gingival bleeding
> ➤ Treatment – corticosteroids, IVIG, platelet transfusion, splenectomy

## *Coagulation Disorders*

1118. What are the most common congenital bleeding and procoagulant/hypercoagulable disorders?

> ➤ Bleeding – von Willebrand's disease (vWD)
> ➤ Procoagulant/hypercoagulable – factor V Leiden

1119. What is the inheritance pattern of vWD?

> ➤ Autosomal dominant

1120. What are the signs and symptoms of vWD?

> ➤ Less severe bleeding – gingival bleeding, epistaxis, heavy menses, prolonged bleeding, petechiae/purpura

1121. What are the treatment options for vWD?

> ➤ DDAVP
> ➤ von Willebrand factor (vWF)/factor 8 concentrates

1122. What is a major clinical manifestation for factor V Leiden?

> VTE (venous thromboembolism)

1123. What is the difference between hemophilia A and B?

> Hemophilia A – lack of factor VIII (8)
> Hemophilia B – lack of factor IX (9)
>   ▪ "Christmas disease"

1124. What is the inheritance pattern of hemophilia?

> X-linked recessive

1125. What are the signs and symptoms of hemophilia?

> More severe bleeding – hemarthrosis, "goose egg," intracranial hemorrhage

1126. What are the treatment options for hemophilia?

> DDAVP
> Clotting factor concentrates

## Thrombocytopenia

1127. What two viral infections must be evaluated for when working up a patient with unexplained thrombocytopenia?

> HIV
> Hepatitis C

1128. What condition is associated with antiphospholipid syndrome? What does it cause? What are some signs and symptoms?

> SLE
> Hypercoagulability
> Recurrent clotting (VTE/DVT/PE), CVA, unexplained pregnancy loss (most likely occurring in the first trimester)

1129. If a patient with purpura appears severely ill, what condition must you consider? What tests must you perform? What common medication rarely causes TTP?

> ➤ Disseminated Intravascular Coagulation (DIC)
> ➤ LFTs and coagulation panels
>   ▪ PT/INR, aPTT, fibrinogen, D-dimer
> ➤ Medication: Clopidogrel

1130. What diagnosis should be considered in a patient with recent IV heparin infusion that presents with purpura?

> ➤ Heparin Induced Thrombocytopenia (HIT)
>   ▪ Test used: HIT antibody (aka heparin-PF4 antibody)

1131. How does Thrombotic Thrombocytopenic Purpura (TTP) present? What blood test is diagnostic? What are the treatment options?

> ➤ Fever, anemia, thrombocytopenia, renal failure, neurologic disturbances
> ➤ Diagnostic lab used: ADAMTS13
> ➤ Treatment – plasmapheresis, high-dose corticosteroids, splenectomy

1132. What are the reversal therapies for Warfarin? Heparin?

> ➤ Warfarin – vitamin K
> ➤ Heparin – protamine sulfate

# Cytopenias

## General

1133. What measurements on the complete blood count (CBC) define anemia if one or more is reduced?

> Hemoglobin, hematocrit, and/or RBC count

1134. What is the process of the formation of all types of blood cells called?

> Hematopoiesis

1135. What is erythropoiesis?

> The production and regulatory process of red blood cells

1136. What causes symptoms of anemia?

> Impaired oxygen delivery to the tissues

1137. What are the most common signs and symptoms of anemia?

> Glossitis, koilonychia, pallor, fatigue, shortness of breath, palpitations, tachycardia

1138. What hemoglobin levels define anemia as defined by the World Health Organizations (WHO)?

> Men: <13 g/dL
> Women: <12 g/dL

1139. What is the most common type of anemia?

> Iron deficiency anemia

1140. What are the two main causes for acute anemia?

> Blood loss
> Hemolysis

1141. What is the significance of an abnormal reticulocyte count?

> Elevated reticulocyte count – functioning bone marrow → hemolysis or bleeding

1142. What are the components of pancytopenia?
> Anemia, thrombocytopenia, and leukopenia

1143. What two nutrient deficiencies are the most common causes of anemia in pregnancy?
> Iron
> Folate

## *Hemolytic Anemia*

1144. What type of anemia should be considered with rapid decrease in hemoglobin concentration and increase in reticulocyte count without acute blood loss?
> Hemolytic anemia

1145. What test would be positive in both warm and cold autoimmune hemolytic anemia?
> Coombs test

1146. What is the first line treatment for warm autoimmune hemolytic anemia?
> Steroids

1147. What is the treatment for cold autoimmune hemolytic anemia?
> Cold avoidance
> Rituximab
> Warmed packed RBCs prior to transfusion
> Plasmapheresis

1148. What are some causes of hemolytic anemia?
> Warm/cold autoimmune hemolytic
> Malignant hematologic cancers
> Certain solid tumor cancers
> PRBC transfusion reaction
> Paroxysmal nocturnal hemoglobinuria (PNH)

> Hereditary spherocytosis
> Thalassemias
> Sickle cell anemia
> G6PD deficiency

1149. What is a neutropenic fever? What is the treatment?

> Fever in a patient with an absolute neutrophil count <500 uL
>  ▪ Common in patients receiving chemotherapy
> Treatment – Sepsis pathway: Antibiotics and IV fluids

## *Macrocytic Anemia*

1150. What is the significance of mean corpuscular volume (MCV)?

> Increased – macrocytic anemia
> Normal – normocytic anemia
> Decreased – microcytic anemia

1151. What are the causes of macrocytic anemia?

> Megaloblastic: Vitamin B12 deficiency, folic acid deficiency
> Non-megaloblastic: Chronic liver disease, alcoholism, bone marrow
> Macrocytosis is also used to determine a patient's compliance with hydroxyurea in sickle cell disease

1152. What are the causes of vitamin B12 deficiency?

> Pernicious anemia – lack of intrinsic factor
> History of gastric surgery
> Vegetarian diet

1153. In patients with chronic alcohol use, what hematologic abnormality is often seen?
 ➤ Macrocytic anemia

1154. What test is used to identify if B12 deficiency is due to pernicious anemia?
 ➤ Schilling test
 ➤ Intrinsic factor antibodies and parietal cell antibodies

1155. What is the difference in presentation between anemia secondary to vitamin B12 deficiency and folic acid deficiency?
 ➤ Vitamin B12 deficiency – neurologic symptoms
 ➤ Folic acid deficiency – no neurologic symptoms

1156. Folate deficiency in pregnancy can lead to what types of birth defects?
 ➤ Neural tube defects

1157. What is the treatment for anemia secondary to vitamin B12 deficiency?
 ➤ PO, IM, or IV vitamin B12
 ➤ If pernicious anemia is diagnosed, patient will require IM cyanocobalamin

1158. What is the treatment for anemia secondary to folic acid deficiency?
 ➤ PO folate

## Normocytic Anemia

1159. What are common causes of normocytic anemia?
 ➤ Acute blood loss
 ➤ Hemolytic anemia
 ➤ Aplastic anemia

> CKD

1160. What is a common genetic disorder that causes episodic hemolytic anemia associated with febrile illnesses and certain medications or foods?

> Glucose-6-phosphate dehydrogenase (G6PD) deficiency

1161. What lab abnormality is associated with aplastic anemia?

> Pancytopenia

1162. Patients with aplastic anemia at increased risk for developing what two hematologic disorders?

> Acute leukemia
> Myelodysplastic syndrome

1163. How is the diagnosis of aplastic anemia confirmed?

> Bone marrow biopsy

## Microcytic Anemia

1164. What are common causes of microcytic anemia?

> Iron deficiency anemia (IDA)
> Lead toxicity
> Anemia of chronic disease (ACD)
> Thalassemias

1165. What labs will be abnormal in IDA?

> Decreased iron/ferritin
> Increased TIBC

1166. What two potential etiologies should be evaluated for first when working up a patient with IDA?

> GI blood loss

> Menstrual blood loss

1167. What is the treatment for IDA?

> Replacement of iron – PO or IV
  - IV iron may be required in patients with history of gastric surgery

1168. What tests should be done to evaluate for occult blood loss or GI malignancy?

> Stool guaiac, colonoscopy

1169. When taking ferrous sulfate, what helps with absorption of the medication? What are common side effects of taking ferrous sulfate?

> Vitamin C or drinking orange juice
> Constipation, dark colored stools, GI upset

1170. What type of anemia does lead poisoning cause?

> Sideroblastic anemia

1171. What are the signs and symptoms of lead toxicity?

> Neurologic symptoms – ataxia, impaired cognition, irritability

1172. What are some causes for anemia of chronic disease (ACD)?

> Chronic kidney disease
> Liver failure/cirrhosis

# Cytoses

## Polycythemia Vera

1173. What are the causes of polycythemia vera (PV)?

> Primary – bone marrow dysfunction

➢ Secondary – chronic hypoxia (COPD), smoking, exogenous erythropoietin use, OSA, high elevations

1174. What are the signs and symptoms of PV?

➢ Headache, visual disturbances, facial plethora, pruritis, hypertension, thrombosis

1175. What labs are abnormal in PV?

➢ Increased hemoglobin/hematocrit and RBC count

1176. What screening is used to detect PV?

➢ JAK2 mutation

1177. What is first line treatment for PV? What is the goal?

➢ Therapeutic phlebotomy
  ▪ Hydroxyurea may be used

➢ Goal: HCT <45%


## *Essential Thrombocytopenia*

1178. What lab value is abnormal in essential thrombocytosis?

➢ Increased platelet count

1179. In essential thrombocytosis (ET), what is the treatment for low-risk and high-risk patients?

➢ Low risk: Aspirin

➢ High risk: Interferon-alpha or hydroxyurea plus aspirin

# Hemoglobinopathies

## Diagnosis

1180. What is the definitive test in the diagnosis of hemoglobinopathies?

> ➤ Hemoglobin electrophoresis

## Hemochromatosis

1181. What is hemochromatosis?

> ➤ Excessive iron absorption which leads to the accumulation of iron in organs

1182. What labs are abnormal in hemochromatosis?

> ➤ Increased iron/ferritin
> ➤ Decreased TIBC

## Sickle Cell Disease

1183. What is the inheritance pattern for sickle cell disease?

> ➤ Autosomal recessive

1184. What are some common complications of sickle cell disease?

> ➤ Vaso-occlusive/aplastic crises (hemolysis)
> ➤ Acute chest syndrome

1185. In which locations does vaso-occlusive pain most commonly occur?

> ➤ Back, chest, abdomen, long bones

1186. How is a patient's pain assessed during an acute vaso-occlusive crisis (VOC)? What is the cornerstone treatment?

> Patient's report of the severity of pain and it's comparison to previous VOCs
> Analgesia – usually requiring opioids
> Hydration
> Supplemental oxygenation

1187. What medication is used to prevent VOC?

> Hydroxyurea

1188. What is dactylitis? Who may present with these symptoms?

> Pain and swelling from infarctions to the soft tissues of the hands and feet
> 6 months to 2 years old during a VOC

## Thalassemia

1189. What are the two types of thalassemia? What do they lead to?

> Alpha thalassemia – defect/absence of the alpha hemoglobin chains
> Beta thalassemia – defect/absence of the beta hemoglobin chains
> Microcytic anemia and hemolysis

1190. What is the treatment of thalassemia?

> Mild to moderate: No treatment
> Severe: RBC transfusion, splenectomy

# Neoplasms

## Leukemias

1191. What is the most common childhood malignancy?

> Acute lymphoblastic leukemia/lymphoblastic lymphoma (ALL/LBL)

1192. What are the most common physical exam findings for children with leukemia?

> Hepatomegaly, splenomegaly, pallor, fever, bruising

1193. What are the three most common leukemias seen with adults?

> Chronic lymphocytic leukemia (CLL)
> Acute myelogenous leukemia (AML)
> Chronic myelogenous leukemia (CML)

1194. What procedure is used to confirm the diagnosis of leukemia?

> Bone marrow aspiration

## *Multiple Myeloma*

1195. What are the five signs and symptoms of multiple myeloma?

> **I**nfection
> hyper**C**alcemia
> **R**enal failure
> **A**nemia
> **B**one disease (ie. lytic lesions, fractures)
  - Remember: "**I CRAB**"

1196. What two findings are present in patients with multiple myeloma requiring therapy?

> Bone marrow clonal plasma cells >10% or biopsy proven plasmacytoma
> Myeloma defining events ("I CRAB" criteria)

## _Hodgkin's & Non-Hodgkin's Lymphoma_

1197. What are the signs and symptoms of both Hodgkin and non-Hodgkin lymphoma?

> ➤ Painless lymphadenopathy and constitutional symptoms (ie. fever, weight loss, fatigue)

# 12

# INFECTIOUS
# DISEASE

# *Bacterial Diseases*

## *Botulism*

1198. What pathogen is responsible for botulism?
  ➤ Clostridium botulinum

1199. What are some common sources of clostridium botulinum?
  ➤ Wound – contaminated soil
  ➤ Food-borne – home-canned goods, preserved or fermented foods
  ➤ Intestinal – honey (infants)

1200. What are the classic signs and symptoms of botulism in an adult?
  ➤ Paralysis and vision abnormalities

1201. What is the classic presentation of botulism in an infant?
  ➤ Floppy infant syndrome

## *Diphtheria*

1202. What pathogen is responsible for diphtheria?
  ➤ Corynebacterium diphtheriae

1203. What are the classic signs and symptoms of diphtheria?
  ➤ Thick grey membrane covering the pharynx (infection of the respiratory tract) and "bull neck"

1204. How is the diagnosis of diphtheria confirmed?
  ➤ Culture from respiratory tract secretions or from cutaneous lesions
  ➤ Positive toxin assay

### *Gonococcal*

1205. How is the risk of contracting gonococcal conjunctivitis reduced in neonates?

> ➤ Prophylactic administration of ophthalmic antibiotic: Erythromycin ophthalmic ointment given immediately after birth

### *MRSA*

1206. What is the treatment for cellulitis or an abscess when there is known or suspected infection due to methicillin-resistant Staphylococcus aureus (MRSA)?

> ➤ Cellulitis: Antibiotics
> ➤ Abscess: Incision & Drainage ± Antibiotics
>> ▪ If MRSA is not suspected, I&D alone may be sufficient

1207. When should parenteral antibiotic therapy be considered when treating MRSA?

> ➤ Failed outpatient PO antibiotic therapy, immunocompromised, extensive soft tissue involvement, sepsis, rapid progression of infection, infection is near/involving an indwelling device

1208. What are common parenteral antibiotics that provide coverage against MRSA?

> ➤ Vancomycin
> ➤ Daptomycin

### *S. Pneumoniae*

1209. What are the four most common clinical manifestations of S. pneumoniae?

Infectious Disease

➤ Pneumonia
➤ Meningitis
➤ Otitis Media (especially in children)
➤ Sinusitis

1210. What intravenous antibiotic is typically used empirically to treat S. Pneumoniae pneumonia in patients admitted to the hospital?
➤ Ceftriaxone

## *Rheumatic Fever*

1211. What is rheumatic fever a complication of?
➤ Group A strep infection

1212. What are the signs and symptoms of rheumatic fever?
➤ Recent strep infection, polyarthritis, carditis, subcutaneous nodules, erythema marginatum, Sydenham's chorea

1213. What criteria is used to diagnose rheumatic fever?
➤ Jones criteria (2 major OR 1 major + 2 minor criteria)
  ▪ Major criteria – "**JONES**"
    • **J**oint involvement
    • my**O**carditis
    • **N**odules
    • **E**rythema marginatum
    • **S**ydenham chorea
  ▪ Minor criteria – "**FLAP**"
    • **F**ever

- <u>L</u>eukocytosis
- <u>A</u>rthralgia
- <u>P</u>rolonged PR interval, increased ESR/CR<u>P</u>, <u>P</u>revious history of rheumatic fever

1214. What antibiotic is used in the treatment of rheumatic fever?

> Penicillin

1215. What cardiac sequelae may develop secondary to rheumatic fever?

> Chronic valvular disorders – most commonly affecting the mitral and aortic valves

## *Rocky Mountain Spotted Fever*

1216. What is the vector for Rocky Mountain spotted fever? What time of the year do most RMSF cases occur?

> Tick species
> Spring and early summer

1217. What organism causes Rocky Mountain Spotted Fever? What is the treatment?

> Organism: Rickettsia rickettsii
> Treatment: Doxycycline

## *Tetanus*

1218. What pathogen is responsible for tetanus?

> Clostridium tetani

1219. Where is Clostridium tetani commonly found? What is the treatment if someone is exposed?

> Contaminated soil
  - Also found in other "dirty" environments

> If they have not had a TDAP in the last 5 years, they can get one post-exposure

1220. What are the signs and symptoms of tetanus?

> Trismus "lockjaw", spasticity, seizures, paralysis

## *Fungal Diseases*
### *Candidal Infections*

1221. What pathogen is responsible for most candidal infections?

> Candida albicans – commonly found in the mouth, throat, GI, vagina, skin

1222. What are some risk factors for candidal infections?

> Immunocompromised (diabetes mellitus, HIV)
> Antibiotic use
> Corticosteroid use
> Pregnancy

## *Mycobacterium Avium Complex*

1223. Which antibiotics are used to treat mycobacterium avium complex (MAC) pneumonia?

> Macrolides (Clarithromycin or Azithromycin)
> Ethambutol
> +/- Rifamycins (Rifampin or Rifabutin)

1224. What pathogen is responsible for TB?

> Mycobacterium tuberculosis

## *Parasitic Diseases*

### *Pinworms*

1225. What is the classic presentation of pinworms?
> Nocturnal perianal pruritis and restless sleep

1226. What test is used to diagnose pinworms?
> Tape test – firmly press the sticky side of clear tape over the anal area overnight to detect eggs

1227. What do roundworm and hookworm both present with? What hematologic abnormality is associated with hookworm?
> GI symptoms (abdominal pain, diarrhea) and cough
> Hookworm - anemia

1228. How does tapeworm present?
> GI symptoms (abdominal pain, loss of appetite) and weight loss

### *Malaria*

1229. What pathogen is responsible for malaria?
> Plasmodium (one-celled parasite)

1230. What is the vector for malaria?
> Mosquito (Anopheles genus)

1231. Which chemoprophylaxis options may be used for malaria prevention?
> Doxycycline, tafenoquine, atovaquone-proguanil, mefloquine

1232. What is the classic presentation of malaria?

> "Flu-like illness" episodes of chills/rigors →
> high fever → diaphoresis following travel to
> tropics/subtropics

1233. What medications are used in the treatment of malaria?

> Antimalarials – chloroquine, artemisinin-based
> combo therapies (ACTs), hydroxychloroquine,
> quinine

## *Giardia*

1234. Who are high-risk populations for Giardia?

> Infants, young children, daycares, travelers,
> international adoptees, immunocompromised

# *Prenatal Transmission of Disorders*

1235. What are examples of infections that may be transmitted during pregnancy and/or birth?

> Varicella
> Rubella
> HSV
> HPV
> CMV
> Zika virus
> Toxoplasmosis
> Hepatitis
> Syphilis
> Gonorrhea
> Chlamydia
> HIV

1236. What are the perinatal infections included in the TORCH acronym?

> **T**oxoplasmosis
> **O**ther (syphilis, varicella, mumps, parvovirus, HIV, parvovirus B19)
> **R**ubella (German measles)
> **C**ytomegalovirus (CMV)
> **H**erpes simplex virus (HSV)

## *Spirochetal Diseases*

### *Lyme Disease*

1237. Which gram-negative bacteria causes Lyme disease? What is the name and appearance of the characteristic rash associated with Lyme disease?

> Borrelia burgdorferi
> Erythema migrans: Bulls-eye morphology
>   • Occurs in up to 90% of cases

1238. What is the treatment for uncomplicated Lyme disease? Complicated Lyme disease?

> Uncomplicated: Doxycycline
> Complicated (i.e. neurological or cardiac involvement): Ceftriaxone

### *Syphilis*

1239. Primary syphilis is characterized by what finding? What symptoms can be present in secondary syphilis? Tertiary syphilis?

> Primary syphilis:
>   • Painless chancre

> Secondary syphilis:
  - Maculopapular rash involving palms/soles
  - Condyloma lata
  - Lymphadenopathy
  - Nonspecific constitutional symptoms (ie. fatigue, fevers, arthralgias)
> Tertiary syphilis:
  - Tabes dorsalis
  - Gummas
  - General paresis
  - Aortitis

1240. What tests are most commonly used for screening (high sensitivity) and confirmation (high specificity) of Syphilis?

> Screening: Rapid plasma regain (RPR), Venereal Disease Research Laboratory (VDRL)
> Confirmation: Fluorescent treponemal antibody absorption (FTA-ABS)

1241. What antibiotic is considered first line for the treatment of syphilis? What is the dosing for early syphilis? For tertiary/late latent syphilis?

> Penicillin G benzathine IM
> Early: 2.4 million units IM once
> Tertiary & Late Latent: 2.4 million units IM weekly for 3 weeks

## Viral Diseases

### Infectious Mononucleosis

1242. What virus causes infectious mononucleosis?

➢ Epstein-Barr virus (EBV)

1243. What is that classic triad of infectious mononucleosis?

➢ Fever, pharyngitis, bilateral posterior cervical lymphadenopathy

1244. What are common symptoms of mononucleosis?

➢ Fatigue, rash (especially after administration of penicillin/amoxicillin for suspected strep pharyngitis), malaise, headache, low grade-fever, splenomegaly

1245. What test is used in the diagnosis of mononucleosis?

➢ Monospot
  ▪ 85% sensitive & 100% specific

1246. What lab abnormality is associated with infectious mononucleosis?

➢ Atypical lymphocytes

1247. What is the treatment for infectious mononucleosis?

➢ Supportive treatment
➢ Rest – avoidance of contact sports for risk of splenic injury/rupture

1248. What is a rare but serious complication of mononucleosis?

➢ Splenomegaly or ruptured spleen

## *HIV/AIDS*

1249. What antibody test is used to screen for HIV? What test is used to confirm HIV?

➢ Screen: ELISA

> Confirm: Western blot

1250. What cells are primarily affected in HIV/AIDS?
> T cells (CD4+)

1251. What CD4 count is diagnostic for AIDS?
> <200

1252. What is the treatment for HIV/AIDS?
> Antiretroviral therapy
> Antibiotic prophylaxis (dependent on CD4 count)
> Prompt treatment of infections

1253. What are physical exam findings that can indicate early HIV infection seen in infants and children?
> Lymphadenopathy
> Hepatosplenomegaly


## Influenza

1254. What type of precautions are recommended to prevent seasonal influenza transmission in the health care setting?
> Droplet precautions


## Measles, Mumps, Rubella (MMR)

1255. What is another name for measles? What is the classic presentation?
> Rubeola
> The "**3 Cs**"
  - **C**ough
  - **C**oryza
  - **C**onjunctivitis + fever
> Koplik spots (buccal mucosa)

> Rash
  ▪ Progresses head → toe

1256. What is the classic presentation of mumps?

> Non-specific viral symptoms (fever, headache, fatigue, muscle ache, loss of appetite)
> Parotitis – parotid gland swelling

1257. Rubella virus is a member in what virus family? What is the classic presentation?

> Family – togaviridae
> Non-specific viral symptoms (low-grade fever, sore throat, rash)
> Lymphadenopathy
> Forschheimer spots – soft palate petechiae
> Rash (head → body)

1258. What is the treatment for measles, mumps, and rubella?

> Symptomatic/supportive treatment

1259. What vaccination prevents measles, mumps, and rubella?

> MMR

## *Erythema Infectiosum*

1260. What is another name for erythema infectiosum? What virus causes it?

> "Fifth Disease"
> Parvovirus B19

1261. How does erythema infectiosum present?

> Non-specific viral symptoms (low-grade fever, malaise)
> "Slapped cheek"

> Rash (maculopapular → lacy reticular) sparing the palms and soles

## Roseola

1262. How does roseola present?
> High fever followed by rash
  - Rash begins on torso and then spreads to the face, arms, and legs

## Rabies

1263. What are some possible vectors for rabies?
> Bats
> Dogs
> Raccoons

1264. What are the signs and symptoms of rabies?
> Pain/paresthesias at site of bite, spasms, paralysis, hypersalivation, coma

1265. What is the prophylaxis/treatment for rabies?
> Immunoglobulin

## Varicella Zoster

1266. What group of individuals should be isolated from a patient with an acute varicella zoster virus (VZV) or herpes zoster virus?
> Pregnant women, immunocompromised patients, unvaccinated

1267. What are the common names for varicella zoster virus? For herpes zoster virus?
> Varicella zoster: Chickenpox
> Herpes zoster: Shingles

1268. How does VZV commonly present?
> Fever and malaise
> Pruritic rash – dew drops on a rose petal, erupt in crops then crust over

1269. What are some possible sequalae of VZV?
> Herpes zoster (shingles)
> Herpes zoster ophthalmicus – Hutchinson's sign
> Herpes zoster oticus – Ramsay-Hunt Syndrome
> Cranial and peripheral nerve palsies
> Meningoencephalitis

1270. What medications may be used to treat VZV if severe infection or if the patient is at risk for complications?
> Antivirals – acyclovir, valcylovir

## Rotavirus

1271. What is the most common cause for severe gastroenteritis worldwide in infants and children?
> Rotavirus

1272. What are common signs/symptoms of rotavirus?
> Diarrhea, vomiting, fever

1273. What are two available rotavirus vaccines? When is their administration recommended?
> RV5 (3 doses): 2, 4, and 6 months old
> RV1 (2 doses): 2 and 4 months old

## Norovirus

1274. What symptoms are associated with norovirus infection?

> Acute onset of vomiting and/or watery diarrhea, abdominal pain

1275. What is an important measure to take for prevention and control of norovirus?

> Hand hygiene by washing with soap and water; virus is not killed with alcohol-based disinfectant

## Zika

1276. What are clinical manifestations of a Zika virus infection?

> Low-grade fever, arthralgia (especially to hands and feet), pruritic maculopapular rash, non-purulent conjunctivitis

1277. What the most common routes of Zika virus transmission?

> Infected mosquito bite
> Maternal-fetal transmission
> Sexual intercourse

1278. What complications are associated with a Zika virus infections?

> Congenital microcephaly
> Fetal loss
> Guillain-Barre syndrome

# Systemic Inflammatory Response Syndrome (SIRS) & Sepsis

1279. How is Systemic Inflammatory Response Syndrome (SIRS) defined?

> ≥2 of the following

- Temperature <36°C (96.8°F) or >38°C (100.4°F)
- HR >90 bpm
- Respiratory rate >20/min or PaCO2 <32 mmHg
- WBC <4,000 or >12,000 or 10% bands

1280. How is sepsis defined?
  ➢ SIRS + source of infection

1281. How is severe sepsis defined?
  ➢ Sepsis + end organ failure (AMS, hypotension, elevated lactate, elevated Cr, elevated LFTs, elevated troponin)

1282. How is septic shock defined?
  ➢ Sepsis + persistent hypotension requiring vasopressors

1283. What laboratory value will be elevated in sepsis?
  ➢ Lactic acid

1284. What should be done prior to administration of antibiotics in sepsis if possible?
  ➢ Blood cultures

1285. What is the treatment for septic shock?
  ➢ Fluid resuscitation – IV fluids
  ➢ Vasopressors – Norepinephrine
  ➢ Initial antimicrobial therapy – IV antibiotics

**13**

# RENAL
# SYSTEM

# *Acute Disorders*

## *General*

1286. What is azotemia?
> ➤ Elevation of BUN, buildup of nitrogenous products
> ➤ May or may not have elevated creatinine levels

1287. What is uremia?
> ➤ Elevated concentrations of urea and other nitrogenous waste products in the blood due to acute kidney injury or renal failure

1288. What is the term used for generalized, gross edema?
> ➤ Anasarca

## *Glomerulonephritis*

1289. Glomerulonephritis (GN) can be divided into what two categories?
> ➤ Nephritic syndrome
> ➤ Nephrotic syndrome

1290. What are clinical manifestations of glomerular disease?
> ➤ Hematuria, proteinuria, renal insufficiency, HTN, edema, hypercoagulability

1291. What is recommended for all patients with glomerulonephritis?
> ➤ Nephrologist consult
> ➤ Kidney biopsy

1292. What are some disorders that may cause nephritic syndrome?

> Post-infectious glomerulonephritis
> IgA nephropathy
> Henoch-Schonlein Purpura (HSP)

1293. What pathogen commonly causes post-infectious glomerulonephritis?

> Streptococcus
  - Post-streptococcal glomerulonephritis (PSGN)

1294. What diagnosis must be considered in a child who presents with abdominal cramping and purpura after a URI?

> Henoch-Schonlein Purpura (HSP)

1295. What are some signs and symptoms of HSP?

> Symmetric purpura in lower extremities, abdominal pain, nephritis, arthritis, edema

1296. What are the signs and symptoms of nephritic syndrome?

> Cola colored urine, oliguria/anuria, edema, hypertension

1297. What lab abnormalities are associated with nephritic syndrome?

> Hematuria, proteinuria (1-3 g/day)

1298. What is seen on urine microscopy in nephritic syndrome? In nephrotic syndrome?

> Nephritic: RBC cast
> Nephrotic: Oval fat bodies

1299. How does nephrotic syndrome commonly present?

> Massive proteinuria (>3.5 g/day), hypoalbuminemia, hyperlipidemia, edema

1300.  What is the most common cause for nephrotic syndrome?
> Diabetic nephropathy

## _Hemolytic Uremic Syndrome_

1301.  What is the triad of manifestations for hemolytic uremic syndrome (HUS)?
> Acute renal failure, hemolytic anemia, & thrombocytopenia

## _Lupus Nephritis_

1302.  What is the most frequent abnormal laboratory finding in patients with lupus nephritis?
> Proteinuria

1303.  How is the diagnosis of lupus nephritis confirmed?
> Kidney biopsy

# _Acute Kidney Injury_

1304. What are the three types of acute kidney injury (AKI)?
> Prerenal – hypoperfusion
> Intrinsic – primary renal toxicity
> Postrenal – obstruction

1305. What are some possible causes of prerenal AKI?
> Dehydration/volume loss
> Third spacing (ie. loss of protein from cirrhosis, renal losses, gastric losses)
> Poor perfusion (ie. heart failure)

1306. What are some possible causes of intrinsic AKI?
  ➢ Acute tubular necrosis (ATN) – ischemia, nephrotoxins
  ➢ Acute interstitial nephritis (AIN) – medications, infection, autoimmune
  ➢ Glomerulonephritis (GN)
  ➢ Vascular disorders

1307. What are some possible causes of postrenal AKI?
  ➢ BPH
  ➢ Urolithiasis
  ➢ Malignancy

1308. What is the most common type of acute renal failure in children?
  ➢ Prerenal (dehydration secondary to diarrhea or vomiting)

1309. What is acute tubular necrosis (ATN)?
  ➢ Severe, prolonged renal hypoperfusion that leads to ischemic injury

1310. What are classic symptoms for rhabdomyolysis?
  ➢ Muscle pain, weakness, dark "coke-appearing" urine

1311. What laboratory test is the hallmark for the diagnosis of rhabdomyolysis?
  ➢ Elevated creatine kinase (CK): Increased at least 5x the upper limit of normal

## Chronic Kidney Disease

1312. What are the most common causes of chronic kidney disease (CKD)?
  ➢ Diabetes

> Hypertension

1313. What measurement is used to stage CKD?

> Glomerular filtration rate (GFR)
  - Stage 1 – ≥90 mL/min
  - Stage 2 – 60-89 mL/min
  - Stage 3 – 30-59 mL/min
  - Stage 4 – 15-29 mL/min
  - Stage 5 – <15 mL/min

1314. When should a patient with chronic kidney disease be referred to a nephrologist?

> GFR is <30 mL/min

1315. What other lab abnormalities may be seen with CKD?

> Increased creatinine and BUN
> Proteinuria
> Anemia
> Hyperkalemia
> Hypermagnesemia
> Hypocalcemia

1316. What medications slow the progression of CKD?

> ACEi/ARBs

1317. What are the most common causes of chronic renal failure in children <5 years old?

> Congenital renal and urinary tract malformations
> Vesicoureteral reflux

1318. What is vesicoureteral reflux? What is the imaging test of choice to diagnosis?

> Retrograde flow of urine from the bladder into the ureters
> Voiding cystourethrogram (VCUG)

# Congenital & Structural Renal Disorders

## Polycystic Kidney Disease

1319. Which autosomal inheritance pattern is most common in polycystic kidney disease in adults? In children?

> Adults: Autosomal dominant
> Children: Autosomal recessive

1320. What are common signs/symptoms of autosomal dominant polycystic kidney disease (ADPKD)?

> Flank pain, abdominal mass, hematuria, UTI, HTN, proteinuria, elevated kidney function

1321. What are risk factors associated with progressive kidney disease in polycystic kidney disease?

> Onset of symptoms at a young age
> Black race
> Male
> Kidney size
> Presence of polycystin-1 mutation
> Hypertension

1322. Since most pediatric patients are with autosomal dominant polycystic kidney disease (ADPKD) are asymptomatic, how is the diagnosis of usually established?

> Positive family history
> Kidney ultrasonography – cysts present

## *Renal Artery Stenosis*

1323. What are some possible causes of renal artery stenosis?

> ➤ Atherosclerosis
> ➤ Fibromuscular dysplasia

1324. What are some common signs and symptoms of renal artery stenosis?

> ➤ Hypertension resistant to drug therapy
> ➤ Increased creatinine/BUN after trial of ACE inhibitor

1325. What is the initial imaging modality used to evaluate for renal artery stenosis?

> ➤ Renal ultrasound

1326. What imaging modality is used to confirm the diagnosis of renal artery stenosis?

> ➤ Renal angiography

1327. What are the surgical treatment options for renal artery stenosis?

> ➤ Renal angioplasty +/- stent
> ➤ Renal artery bypass

## *End-Stage Renal Disease*

1328. What are signs/symptoms of uremia?

> ➤ Fatigue, pruritis, anorexia, nausea, vomiting, AMS

1329. What GFR is indicative of end-stage renal disease (ESRD)?

> ➤ Stage 5 – <15 mL/min

1330. What are the treatment options for patients with end-stage renal disease (ESRD)?

> Hemodialysis – AV fistula, AV graft, indwelling catheter
> Peritoneal dialysis
> Kidney transplant

1331. When should a patient receive emergent dialysis?

> **A**cidosis (pH <7.1, unable to correct with other resuscitation)
> **E**lectrolytes (K >6.5 mEq/L not responding to treatment or rapidly increasing; hypercalcemia)
> **I**ngestions (methanol, ethylene glycol, lithium, salicylates)
> **O**verload (Volume overload unresponsive to diuresis, CHF)
> **U**remia (Elevated BUN with signs of uremia like bleeding, pericarditis, encephalopathy)
  - Remember: "**AEIOU**"

## *Fluid & Electrolyte Disorders*

### *General*

1332. What pH correlates with acidosis?
> pH <7.35

1333. What pH correlates with alkalosis?
> pH >7.45

1334. What component of the acid-base balance is related to metabolic pathology?

> Bicarbonate ($HCO_3$)
  - Increased $HCO_3$ = metabolic alkalosis
  - Decreased $HCO_3$ = metabolic acidosis

1335. What organ is bicarbonate ($HCO_3$) produced by?

➤ Kidneys

1336. Is bicarbonate ($HCO_3$) an acid or a base?

➤ Base

1337. What is the normal range for bicarbonate ($HCO_3$)?

➤ 22-26 mEq/L

1338. What component of the acid-base balance is related to respiratory pathology?

➤ Carbon dioxide ($pCO_2$)

- Increased $pCO_2$ = respiratory acidosis
- Decreased $pCO_2$ = respiratory alkalosis

1339. What organ produces carbon dioxide ($pCO_2$)?

➤ Lungs

1340. Is carbon dioxide ($pCO_2$) an acid or a base?

➤ Acid

1341. What is the normal range for carbon dioxide ($pCO_2$)?

➤ 35-45 mmHg

1342. What are the most common causes of elevated anion gap metabolic acidosis?

➤ **M**ethanol

➤ **U**remia

➤ **D**KA

➤ **P**aracetamol (acetaminophen)

➤ **I**ron/**I**soniazid

➤ **L**actic acidosis

➤ **E**thylene glycol

➤ **S**alicylates

- Remember: "**MUDPILES**"

1343. What are the most common causes of non-anion gap metabolic acidosis?
  - ➤ **H**yperalimentation (TPA)
  - ➤ **A**cetazolamide/**A**mphotericin
  - ➤ **R**ental tubular acidosis
  - ➤ **D**iarrhea
  - ➤ **U**reteral diversion
  - ➤ **P**ancreatic fistula
    - ▪ Remember: "**HARD UP**"

1344. What are common causes of metabolic alkalosis?
  - ➤ Vomiting
  - ➤ Diuresis

1345. What are common causes of respiratory acidosis?
  - ➤ Hypoventilation
  - ➤ Pulmonary disease

1346. What are common causes of respiratory alkalosis?
  - ➤ Hyperventilation
  - ➤ Anxiety

1347. What is the most common cause of hyperkalemia?
  - ➤ Acute onset renal dysfunction

1348. What serious clinical manifestations may occur with a serum potassium is ≥7.0 mEq/L?
  - ➤ Muscle weakness or paralysis, cardiac arrhythmias

1349. What is the classic EKG finding seen with hyperkalemia?
  - ➤ Peaked T-waves

1350. What are the treatment options for hyperkalemia?

> Calcium
> Sodium bicarbonate
> Insulin/dextrose
> Kayexalate
> Albuterol
> Furosemide
> Dialysis

1351. What is the treatment for hypokalemia?

> PO or IV potassium

1352. What other electrolyte abnormality is associated with hypokalemia?

> Hypomagnesemia

1353. What protein must be accounted for when calculating corrected calcium?

> Albumin

1354. What are the treatment options for hypercalcemia?

> IV fluids
> Calcitonin
> IV bisphosphonates
> Loop diuretics
> Dialysis

1355. What are hallmark symptoms of severe hypocalcemia?

> Tetany: Peripheral neuromuscular irritability, muscle cramps, paresthesias of hands and feet, carpopedal spams

1356. What is the treatment for hypocalcemia?

> Mild: Calcium Carbonate or Calcium Citrate

> Severe: IV Calcium Gluconate

1357. What are the common causes of hypermagnesemia?

> Iatrogenic

> Laxative/enema use

> Renal failure

1358. What are the treatment options for hypermagnesemia?

> Calcium

> IV NS/furosemide

> Dialysis

1359. What are the common causes of hypomagnesemia?

> Alcohol abuse

> IBD

> Endocrine disorders

> Decreased PO intake

1360. What cardiac arrhythmia does hypomagnesemia cause?

> Torsades de pointes (TdP)

1361. What is the treatment for hypomagnesemia?

> IV magnesium

1362. What is the treatment for hypernatremia? What are some causes of hypernatremia? What are common symptoms of hypernatremia?

> IV NS

> Causes: Lack of water, diuretics, osmotic losses from hyperglycemia, GI losses, diabetes insipidus, nephrogenic diabetes insipidus

> Symptoms: Lethargy, weakness, irritability
  ▪ These may progress to coma or death

1363. What is the complication associated with correcting hypernatremia too quickly?

> Cerebral edema

1364. What are the three types of hyponatremia?

> Hypovolemic
> Euvolemic
> Hypervolemic

1365. What are common causes of hypertonic hyponatremia (pseudohyponatremia)?

> Hyperglycemia, hyperlipidemia, hyperproteinemia

1366. In a patient with acute symptomatic hyponatremia what should be the maximum rate of correction?

> Sodium correction should not exceed 8 mEq/L/d

1367. When is hypertonic saline used in hyponatremia?

> AMS or seizures with sodium <120 mEq/L

1368. What is the complication associated with correcting hyponatremia too quickly?

> Central pontine myelinolysis

## *SIADH*

1369. What disorder causes inappropriate water retention due to an inability to suppress the secretion of antidiuretic hormone (ADH)?

> Syndrome of inappropriate secretion of antidiuretic hormone (SIADH)

1370. What are the common causes of syndrome of inappropriate diuretic hormone (SIADH)?

➤ Stroke, brain trauma, antipsychotics, antidepressants, cancer, pneumonia, pain, surgery

1371. What are common lab findings seen with SIADH?

➤ Hyponatremia
➤ Decreased serum osmolality (<280 mOsm/kg)
➤ Increased urine osmolality (>100 mOsm/kg)
➤ Urine sodium concentration >40 mEq/L

1372. What are initial treatments of hyponatremia in SIADH?

➤ Treat the underlying disease
➤ Initiate therapy to increase serum sodium levels
➤ Fluid restriction (mainstay therapy) with goal intake of <800 mL/day

# Renal System

# 14

# MUSCUOLOSKELETAL SYSTEM

## Chest & Rib Disorders

1373. What is the difference between pectus excavatum and pectus carinatum?

> Pectus excavatum – concave deformity of the anterior chest wall

> Pectus carinatum – convex deformity of the anterior chest wall

1374. What is flail chest? What classic sign is seen with respiration? What injury is it commonly associated with?

> ≥2 contiguous rib fractures with each rib broken in ≥2 places

> Paradoxical movement of the chest wall

> Underlying pulmonary contusion

## Compartment Syndrome

1375. What lower extremity fracture is most commonly associated with compartment syndrome? What compartment does it most commonly affect?

> Tibial shaft fracture

> Anterior leg compartment

1376. What are the classic symptoms of compartment syndrome?

> **P**ain (out of proportion with passive ROM)

> **P**allor

> **P**aresthesias

> **P**oikilothermia

> **P**ulselessness

> **P**aralysis

- Remember: "**6 P's**"

1377. What intercompartmental pressure is diagnostic of compartment syndrome? What is the treatment?

> ≥30 mmHg
> Delta pressure <30 mmHg
- Difference between measured compartment pressure and diastolic blood pressure
> Treatment – emergent fasciotomy

## *Osteoarthritis*

1378. What are the classic signs/symptoms of osteoarthritis?

> Joint pain and stiffness that is worse with activity and better with rest
> Heberden's nodes (DIP) and Bouchard's nodes (PIP) – hand OA
> No systemic symptoms or extraarticular findings

1379. What are risk factors for osteoarthritis?

> Aging, obesity, history of intraarticular injury, genetics, females > males, previous orthopedic surgery

1380. What would you see on x-ray in a patient with osteoarthritis?

> Asymmetric joint space narrowing
> Osteophytes
> Subchondral sclerosis
> Subchondral cysts

1381. What are the treatment options for osteoarthritis?

- NSAIDs/Acetaminophen
- Activity modification
- PT
- Intraarticular corticosteroid injections
- Surgery (joint replacement)

1382. Which populations of patients should avoid NSAIDs?

- ≥60 years of age
- History of GI bleeding
- Cardiovascular disease
- Kidney disease
- Aspirin sensitivity syndrome
- Chronic liver disease, hepatic cirrhosis
- Pregnancy

## *Osteoporosis*

1383. What is osteoporosis?

- Bone disease characterized by decreased bone mineral density and bone mass, resulting in increased risk of fractures

1384. What lifestyle measures can be taken in postmenopausal women to reduce bone loss?

- Adequate calcium and vitamin intake, regular exercise, smoking cessation, avoidance of heavy alcohol use, fall prevention

1385. Which class of medication may increase bone loss?

- Glucocorticoids

1386. What is the recommended adequate intake of calcium for postmenopausal women? Vitamin D?

➤ Calcium: 1200 mg daily
➤ Vitamin D: 800 IU daily

1387. What tool is available to help diagnosis osteoporosis and assess for bone mineral density changes?

➤ Dual-energy x-ray absorptiometry (DEXA)

1388. What are the definitions of osteopenia and osteoporosis based upon T-scores?

➤ Osteopenia: T-score between -1 and -2.5
➤ Osteoporosis: T-score <-2.5

1389. Which medications are considered first line treatments in osteoporosis?

➤ Bisphosphonates
➤ Vitamin D

## Rickets

1390. What is the daily recommended intake of vitamin D for infants?

➤ 400 IU daily
➤ Exclusively breastfed infants will need
   supplementation

1391. What conditions can occur in infants and children with severe vitamin D deficiency?

➤ Rickets

## Infectious Diseases
### Osteomyelitis

1392. What is the most common organism responsible for both osteomyelitis and septic arthritis?

➢ S. aureus

1393. What organism is associated with osteomyelitis of the foot following a puncture wound through the shoe? What antibiotic is used as prophylaxis in this scenario?

➢ Pseudomonas

➢ Ciprofloxacin

1394. When radiographs are normal in a patient with a diabetic foot infection, when should MRI be considered to further assess for osteomyelitis?

➢ Bone is grossly visible or probed

➢ Ulcer >2 cm or present for >1-2 weeks

➢ ESR >70

## Septic Joint

1395. What organism should be considered in a patient <35 years old with septic arthritis?

➢ Neisseria gonorrhoeae

1396. What are the most commonly affected joints in septic arthritis? What is the best diagnostic test for septic arthritis? Which labs should be ordered in the setting of an infection?

➢ Knee > hip > shoulder > elbow > ankle

➢ Joint aspiration with synovial fluid analysis

➢ CBC with differential, ESR, CRP

1397. What would be seen on synovial fluid analysis in a patient with septic arthritis?

➢ WBC >50,000

➢ >75% PMNs

1398. What are complications of a joint injection?

➤ Septic joint, septic bursitis, tendon rupture,
neurovascular damage, bleeding, allergic reactions

1399. What condition is a relative contraindication to
performing a joint aspiration?

➤ Skin or soft tissue infection overlying the area of
the aspiration

## *Tenosynovitis*

1400. What are the Kanavel cardinal signs seen with
infectious flexor tenosynovitis?

➤ Tenderness on the flexor tendon sheath
➤ Slight flexion of finger at rest
➤ Pain with passive extension
➤ Fusiform swelling of the digit "sausage" digit

# *Upper Extremity Disorders*

## *Clavicle*

1401. Which part of the clavicle is most commonly
fractured? What is the treatment in a fracture without
significant shortening and displacement?

➤ Middle third
➤ Nonoperative, sling immobilization

## *Shoulder*

1402. What is the most common type of shoulder
dislocation? What is the typical mechanism of injury?

➤ Anterior
➤ Opposing force when arm is abducted,
extended, and externally rotated

- Example: Being blocked while shooting a basketball

1403. What are the most common causes of a posterior shoulder dislocation?

➤ Electrocution
➤ Seizures
  - Internal rotators of the shoulder (pectoralis muscles) overpower the external rotators

1404. What are the muscles of the rotator cuff? Which physical exam tests are used to evaluate each of them?

➤ **S**upraspinatus – empty can, drop arm
➤ **I**nfraspinatus – external rotation
➤ **T**eres minor – horn blower's
➤ **S**ubscapularis – belly press, lift off
  - Remember: "**SITS**"

1405. What underlying disorders are commonly associated with adhesive capsulitis? What would be seen on physical exam?

➤ Diabetes mellitus and hypothyroidism
➤ Loss of active and passive shoulder ROM (most notably in ER)

## *Elbow*

1406. What radiographic finding on a lateral elbow x-ray is consistent with an occult fracture?

➤ Posterior fat pad – always abnormal
  - Anterior fat pad may be a normal finding if the elbow is flexed

1407. What is a nursemaid's elbow? What is the most common mechanism of injury?

➢ Subluxation of the radial head under the annular ligament

➢ Sudden traction of an extended arm, commonly associated with swinging a child or lifting by one arm

1408. What are the two methods for reduction of a nursemaid's elbow?

➢ Supination/flexion technique

➢ Hyperpronation technique

1409. What physical exam sign is associated with a proximal bicep tendon rupture?

➢ "Popeye" deformity

1410. What are the common names for medial and lateral epicondylitis? What physical exam maneuvers are used to assess for each?

➢ Medial epicondylitis (golfer's elbow) – resisted wrist flexion and pronation

➢ Lateral epicondylitis (tennis elbow) – resisted wrist/middle finger extension

## *Forearm*

1411. What is the difference between a greenstick and a buckle/torus fracture?

➢ Greenstick – incomplete fracture with failure along the tension (convex) side, plastic deformation

➢ Buckle/torus – incomplete, unicortical compression fracture

### Hand & Wrist

1412. What is a Colles' fracture? Smith's fractures?
> Colles' – dorsally angulated distal radius fracture
> Smith's – volarly angulated distal radius fracture

1413. Tenderness in the anatomical snuffbox is suggestive of what fracture?
> Scaphoid fracture

1414. If there is a high suspicion for a scaphoid fracture, but negative x-rays, what is the appropriate management? Why?
> Thumb spica cast or splint and follow-up x-ray in 14-21 days
> High-risk for AVN

1415. What is a boxer's fracture?
> Fracture of the 5th metacarpal neck

1416. What is the classic presentation of a ganglion cyst? What is the treatment?
> Soft, nontender mass on dorsum of wrist that transilluminates
> Treatment
  - Asymptomatic – observation
  - Symptomatic – aspiration, corticosteroid injection, or surgical resection (high rate of recurrence)

1417. What physical exam maneuver is used in the diagnosis of DeQuervain's tenosynovitis? What is the first line of treatment?
> Finkelstein's test – ulnar deviation of the wrist with thumb held in closed first

> Conservative care – rest, NSAIDs, thumb spica splint
>> ▪ May consider steroid injection if symptoms continue

## *Lower Extremity Disorders*

### *Hip*

1418. What are some common causes of avascular necrosis (AVN) of the hip?
> ➤ Alcohol abuse
> ➤ Chronic steroid use
> ➤ Sickle cell disease
> ➤ History of hip dislocation/fracture/surgery
> ➤ Cigarette smoking

1419. What initial diagnostic study should be obtained in a patient with suspected osteonecrosis of the hip?
> ➤ Plain radiography

1420. What is the most common cause of hip pain in a pediatric patient that is associated with history of a recent upper respiratory infections in the absence of fever, elevation in WBC, ESR, or CRP? What is the treatment?
> ➤ Transient synovitis
> ➤ Anti-inflammatory medications (Toradol challenge)

1421. What is developmental dysplasia of the hip (DDH)? What are some risk factors?
> ➤ Abnormal acetabular development resulting in a shallow socket with femoral head subluxation or dislocation

> Risk Factors:
>   - **F**irst born
>   - **F**emale
>   - **F**rank breech
>   - **F**amily history
>     - Remember: "**4 F's**"

1422. What two physical exam maneuvers are used to test for DDH?

> - Barlow – adduction and depression of the femur (dislocates the hip)
> - Ortolani – abduction and elevation of the femur (reduces dislocated hip)

1423. What is the Galeazzi sign?

> - Limb length discrepancy noted at the top of the knees when patient is supine with hips and knees flexed to 90°

1424. What imaging modalities are used to screen for DDH?

> - <4 months – ultrasound
> - >4 months – x-ray
>   - Femoral head begins to ossify at 4 months of age

1425. What is the treatment for DDH in a patient <6 months old?

> - Pavlik harness

1426. What is the Salter-Harris fracture classification for pediatric fractures?

> - Type I – **S**traight through the physis
> - Type II – Traverses the physis, exits in metaphysis (**A**bove)

> Type III – Traverses the physis, exits in epiphysis (**B**elow)
> Type IV – Involves the metaphysis, physis, and epiphysis (**T**hrough)
> Type V – Crush injury to the physis (**R**ammed)
   - Remember: "**SALTeR**"

1427. What is the classic presentation of trochanteric bursitis? What is the treatment?

> Lateral hip pain/tenderness that is worse at night when lying on affected hip
> PT, NSAIDs, cortisone injection

1428. What direction of hip dislocation is most common? How will the lower extremity appear following this type of dislocation?

> Posterior
> Leg shortened, adducted, and internally rotated

1429. Following a native hip dislocation, why should a CT scan of the hip be ordered following reduction?

> To evaluate for acetabular or femoral head fractures, loose bodies, marginal impaction, and joint congruency

1430. How will the lower extremity appear following a hip fracture?

> Leg shortened and externally rotated

1431. What test should be ordered to evaluated for occult hip fracture if clinical suspicion is high with a negative plain radiograph?

> MRI (most sensitive) or CT scan

## *Pelvis*

1432. What potentially fatal complication should be monitored for following a pelvic fracture?

> ➤ Hemorrhage

## *Knee*

1433. What is Osgood-Schlatter disease? How does it present? What is the treatment?

> ➤ Tibial tubercle apophysitis that commonly occurs in adolescent boys who participate in sports that involve running or jumping
> ➤ Anterior knee pain and swelling that is worse with activity and relieved with rest
> ➤ Activity modification, ice/heat, NSAIDs, bracing

1434. Are medial or lateral meniscal injuries more common? How do patients typically present? What positive physical exam tests are highly suggestive of this pathology? What imaging should be obtained?

> ➤ Medial
> ➤ Mechanical symptoms (locking, clicking, catching, popping), joint line tenderness
> ➤ McMurray's, Apley's Compression Test
> ➤ MRI

1435. How do ACL injuries classically present? What physical exam tests are used to diagnose them? What imaging should be obtained?

> ➤ Non-contact twisting mechanism, audible "pop," immediate swelling (hemarthrosis)

➢ Lachman's (most sensitive), anterior drawer, pivot shift

➢ MRI

1436. Which ligaments does a posterior drawer sign assess?

➢ Posterior drawer sign: posterior cruciate ligament (PCL)

1437. Where is a Baker's cyst located? What are common signs/symptoms?

➢ Popliteal region

➢ Posterior knee pain, swelling or palpable mass behind knee, knee stiffness

1438. What is the common name for medial tibial stress syndrome? What is the treatment?

➢ Shin splints

➢ Treatment: Rest (ie. stop physical activity for several weeks), ice, NSAIDS, elevate extremities

## Foot & Ankle

1439. What physical exam tool can be used to help determine if x-ray imaging is warranted for foot and ankle injuries?

➢ Ottawa Ankle Rule

1440. What is a Lisfranc injury? What is the classic physical exam finding?

➢ Tarsometatarsal fracture dislocation between medial cuneiform and base of the second metatarsal

▪ Isolated ligamentous injury may occur with a fracture

Musculoskeletal System

➢ Plantar ecchymosis

1441. What is the difference between a Jones fracture and a pseudo-Jones fracture? How are they treated?

➢ Jones fracture – fracture at the base of the 5<sup>th</sup> metatarsal at the metaphyseal diaphyseal junction
- Treatment – non-weight bearing with short leg splint/cast, surgery in athletes
➢ Pseudo-Jones fracture – proximal tubercle avulsion fracture of the 5<sup>th</sup> metatarsal
- Treatment – protected weight bearing with stiff soled shoe/walking boot

1442. Which ligaments are injured with inversion and eversion ankle injuries?

➢ Inversion – lateral
- Anterior talofibular ligament (ATFL), Calcaneofibular ligament (CFL), and Posterior talofibular ligament (PTFL)
➢ Eversion – medial
- Deltoid ligament

1443. What class of antibiotics is associated with Achilles tendon rupture? What positive physical exam test is highly suggestive of this pathology? What is the treatment?

➢ Fluoroquinolones
➢ Thompson test – with patient lying prone, squeezing of the calf should cause ankle plantarflexion. If the achilles is torn, no ankle plantarflexion is observed
➢ Serial casting (20-30° plantarflexion), boot with heel lift, or surgical repair

1444. What is hallux valgus?
> Bunion – valgus deformity of the MTP of the great toe (plantarflexed and pronated)

1445. How does plantar fasciitis most commonly present? What are the treatment options?
> Pain in the heel of the foot that is worse with the first steps in the morning and after prolonged standing
> Stretching/massage, orthotics, NSAIDs, PT, corticosteroid injections, surgery

## Neoplasms

1446. What signs and symptoms are concerning for bone neoplasm?
> Pain at night (especially if it wakes from sleep), fever/chills, fatigue, weight loss, palpable mass, pathologic fracture

1447. What is osteoid osteoma? What are the common clinical findings?
> Benign bone-forming tumor
> Usually lower extremity pain (proximal femur most common site), increased pain that is worse at night and relived with NSAIDs

1448. Which bone neoplasm occurs in children and young adults and often mimics an infection?
> Ewing sarcoma

# Rheumatologic Disorders

## Systemic Lupus Erythematosus (SLE)

1449. What are the signs and symptoms of Systemic Lupus Erythematosus (SLE)?

> ➢ **S**erositis (pericarditis, pleuritis)
> ➢ **O**ral ulcers
> ➢ **A**rthritis
> ➢ **P**hotosensitivity
> ➢ **B**lood disorders
> ➢ **R**enal disease
> ➢ **A**NA positive
> ➢ **I**mmunologic (anti-Sm, anti-dsDNA)
> ➢ **N**eurologic disorders
> ➢ **M**alar rash
> ➢ **D**iscoid rash
>> ▪ Remember: "**<u>SOAP BRAIN MD</u>**"

1450. What are the treatment options for SLE?

> ➢ NSAIDs
> ➢ Corticosteroids
> ➢ Hydroxychloroquine
> ➢ Methotrexate

## Rheumatoid Arthritis (RA)

1451. What are the classic signs and symptoms of rheumatoid arthritis (RA)?

> ➢ Bilateral joint pain and stiffness that is better with activity and worse with rest (MCP, PIP; DIP spared)

➤ Swan neck and Boutonniere deformities – hand RA
➤ Systemic symptoms (fever, fatigue)
➤ Extraarticular findings (skin, heart, lungs, kidneys, eyes)

1452. What lab markers are associated RA?
➤ Increased ESR/CRP
➤ Positive RF
➤ Positive Anti-CCP (most specific)

1453. What are the treatment options for RA?
➤ NSAIDs
➤ PT
➤ Corticosteroids
➤ Disease Modifying Anti-Rheumatic Drugs (DMARDs) – methotrexate, hydroxychloroquine, sulfasalazine
➤ Biologics
➤ Surgery

1454. What is the name for the condition that presents with joint pain, extraarticular symptoms, and increased ESR/CRP in a child <16-years-old? What are the different types of this condition?
➤ Juvenile Rheumatoid Arthritis/Juvenile Idiopathic Arthritis (JIA)
➤ Systemic/Still's disease, Pauciarticular, and Polyarticular

## Sjogren's Syndrome

1455. What are the signs/symptoms of Sjögren's syndrome? What tests are used to diagnose it?

> Dry mucous membranes (eyes, mouth, vagina), excessive thirst, joint pain
> Schirmer test and lip biopsy

## *Polymyalgia Rheumatica*

1456. What are the classic symptoms of Polymyalgia Rheumatica (PMR)? What condition commonly occurs with it?

> Proximal muscle pain and stiffness (no muscle weakness), low-grade fever, anemia, fatigue
> Giant cell arteritis (GCA)

## *Reactive Arthritis*

1457. What is another name for reactive arthritis? What are some common causes?

> Reiter's syndrome
> Sexually transmitted infection (chlamydia) or food-borne illness (salmonella, campylobacter, shigella, yersinia)

1458. What are the signs and symptoms of reactive arthritis?

> Conjunctivitis
> Urethritis
> Arthritis
  - Remember: "Can't see, can't pee, can't climb a tree"

## *Raynaud's Syndrome*

1459. What is Raynaud's syndrome? How does it present? What is the treatment?

> Vasospasm that causes reduced blood flow to the distal extremity
> Distal extremity pain and skin changes (white → blue → red) following exposure to cold temperatures
> Treatment – avoid cold temperatures, vasodilators (calcium channel blockers)

## Gout

1460. What is the "classic" location for gouty attacks? What is gout in this location called?

> First MTP joint
> Podagra

1461. What are some common risk factors for gout?

> Diet high in purines (meat and seafood) and alcohol use
> Hydrochlorothiazide use

1462. What is the difference between gout and pseudogout crystals on microscopy?

> Gout (monosodium urate) – needle-shaped, negatively birefringent
> Pseudogout (calcium pyrophosphate) – rhomboid-shaped, positively birefringent

1463. What medications are used to treat an acute flare of gout or pseudogout?

> NSAIDs (indomethacin)
> Oral steroids (consider when NSAIDs are contraindicated)
> Colchicine
> Corticosteroid injection

1464. What is the first line preventative medication for gout?

  ➤ Allopurinol

## *Fibromyalgia*

1465. How does fibromyalgia typically present?

  ➤ Extraarticular pain and tenderness that occurs in 11/18 trigger points in addition to sleep/cognitive disturbances in a patient with a history of a rheumatologic disorder, IBS, anxiety, depression

## *Spinal Disorders*

1466. Who does ankylosing spondylitis (AS) most commonly affect? What are the signs and symptoms? What physical exam test is used as part of the diagnosis?

  ➤ Young adult/middle-aged men
  ➤ Ascending back pain and stiffness that begins at the SI joint, decreased chest wall expansion, uveitis
  ➤ Schober test – measures lumbar spine flexion

1467. What are the most common signs and symptoms of cauda equina syndrome? What is the diagnostic test of choice? What is the treatment?

  ➤ Bowel/bladder dysfunction (urinary retention, overflow incontinence, bowel incontinence), loss of anal sphincter tone, saddle paresthesias, leg pain/paresthesias, and leg weakness
  ➤ MRI

> Emergent surgical decompression

1468. What is a positive straight leg raise (SLR) test? What does it indicate?

> Pain radiating below the knee that occurs with passive hip flexion beyond 30° when the patient is lying in the supine position with the knee fully extended

> Lumbar radiculopathy

1469. What defines thoracic kyphosis?

> >40° convex curvature of the thoracic spine

1470. What is scoliosis? How is it named?

> ≥10° lateral curvature of the spine

> Named for the side of convexity

■ Think of it as an arrow pointing towards the named side on a PA radiograph

1471. What tests are used in the diagnosis of scoliosis?

> Adam's forward bend – scoliometer reading of 7°-20° spinal curvature

> X-ray – Cobb angle ≥10°

1472. What is the treatment for scoliosis based on degree of curvature?

> 10-24° – observation

> 25-49° – bracing

> ≥50° – surgery

1473. What is the classic presentation of spinal stenosis?

> Leg/back pain that is worse with walking and extension of the spine and relieved with flexion of the spine (shopping cart sign)

1474. What are some "red flags" for a patient with back pain?

> \>50 years old, immunosuppression, IV drug use, chronic steroid use, trauma, fever, history of cancer, saddle anesthesia, loss of bowel or bladder, weakness, syncope, unexplained weight loss, history of invasive epidural/spine procedure

1475. What are some "red flags" physical exam findings in a patient with back pain?

> Saddle anesthesia, urinary retention, loss of rectal tone, abnormal vital signs (tachycardic, fever, hypotensive, hypoxic), pulse deficits, motor weakness, abnormal deep tendon reflexes, pain on palpation to spinous processes

1476. What is the treatment for a lumbar strain?

> Short-term rest followed by gradual return to activity
> Ice/heat
> NSAIDs
> PT

1477. How does torticollis present? What muscle is contracted?

> Limited neck ROM – most commonly flexed to one side and rotated to the contralateral side
> Sternocleidomastoid muscle (SCM)

1478. What is spondylolysis? What sports may predispose patients to this injury? What radiographic sign is seen on oblique xrays?

> Anatomic defect of the pars interarticularis

> Gymnastics, diving, football, rowing
  (hyperextension sports)
> Scotty dog sign

1479. What is spondylolisthesis?

> Forward translation of one vertebral segment
  relative to the next caudal segment

1480. What is neurogenic shock? What vital signs are typically seen?

> Spinal cord dysfunction secondary to trauma
  that leads to loss of sympathetic tone
> Hypotension and bradycardia

1481. What is the best imaging test to diagnosis a herniated disk?

> MRI

1482. What are the Nexus Criteria that must be present to clinically clear a low-risk patient from cervical spine fracture without obtaining imaging of cervical spine?

> <60 years old
> No posterior midline cervical spine tenderness
> No altered mental status
> No focal neurologic deficits
> No evidence of intoxication
> No painful distracting injuries (long bone
  fractures, crush injuries, large body surface burns,
  visceral injury needing surgical consult, large
  lacerations)

# 15

## HEALTHCARE POLICY & ETHICS

## *General*

1483. What is an advanced directive? A living will?

> Advanced directive: Written statement outlining the patient's health care wishes

> Living will: Written statement outlining the wishes of an individual should they be unable to make their own decisions
>   - A type of advanced directive
>   - Used primarily with the terminally ill

1484. Who is a healthcare power of attorney?

> An individual appointed by the patient to make the patient's healthcare decisions should the patient become incapacitated

1485. Who enforces the Health Insurance Portability and Accountability Act (HIPPA)? What are the four main HIPPA components?

> The Office of Civil Rights

> Privacy Rule, Security Rule, Enforcement Rule, Breach Notification Rule

1486. What are the three main goals of the Affordable Care Act (ACA)?

> To make health insurance more affordable to more people, especially for individuals and small-group purchasers

> To expand Medicaid coverage to adults with incomes below 138% of the Federal Poverty Level

> Encouraged and support medical care delivery methods that are aimed at lowering costs of health care

1487. What are the goals of a root cause analysis?
> Improvement of patient safety
> Preventing future harm
> Identify prevention strategies

1488. What is an unexpected event in a healthcare setting that results in death, serious physical or psychological injury?
> Sentinel event

1489. What is the process when the health care provider communicates and educates the patient about the risks, benefits, and alternatives for a medical procedure or intervention called?
> Informed consent

1490. What is nonmaleficence? What is beneficence?
> Nonmaleficence: The obligation to do no harm
> Beneficence: To do good and not harm

1491. What term refers to the ethical principle of being fair to all individuals?
> Justice

1492. What term refers to being faithful, loyal, and honoring promises in a relationship?
> Fidelity

1493. What term refers to telling the truth and providing the patient with all accurate information?
> Veracity

1494. What is the ethical principle called when a mentally competent adult patient has the right to make informed decisions about their own medical care and treatment?
> Autonomy

1495. What is utilitarianism?

> The obligation to do whatever produces the greatest good for the majority

1496. What is needed to establish a medical malpractice case?

> Duty of care: Provider-patient relationship was established

> Breach of the standard of care

> Causation/Injury

> Proof of damages

1497. What is the difference between medical negligence and medical malpractice?

> Medical negligence: An unintentional act of carelessness, not intended to cause harm

> Medical malpractice: Harm is caused when a provider knowingly fails to meet the standards of care

1498. What criteria is used to measure whether negligence has occurred?

> Standards of care

1499. What three components must be present for a patient to be able to refuse treatment or leave against medical advice, even if it may lead to death?

> Patient has received all information to make an informed decision

> Patient must be of legal age to consent

> Patient must be mentally component to understand the information

1500. What are examples of when minors can seek medical treatment without having the consent from their parents?

> Pregnancy, STIs, drug/alcohol treatment, contraceptives

# <u>Notes</u>

# <u>Notes</u>

# Notes

# <u>Notes</u>

# <u>Notes</u>

# <u>Notes</u>

# Notes

# <u>Notes</u>

# Notes